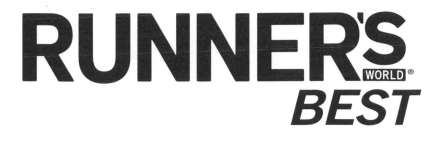

# RUNNER'S WORLD® BEST

# GETTING STARTED

EDITED BY ADAM BEAN,
*RUNNER'S WORLD®* MAGAZINE

RODALE®

D0102969

First published in 2006 by Rodale International Ltd., London, England

© 2006 by Rodale Inc.

Interior photographs: Brand X Pictures: 94; Comstock: 19, 67, 72; Corbis: 58; Digital Vision: 15, 28, 31, 36, 52, 57, 79; Eyewire: 60; Image Source: 38, 49; © 2006 JupiterImages Corporation: 25; LLC, Fogstock: 17, 77, 91; MedioImages: 22; Michael Mazzeo: 40, 41, 42, 43, 44, 45; Photodisk: 18, 35, 74, 84; photolibrary. com pty.ltd.: 70; Pixtal: 86; Rodale Photo Library: 6, 9, 10, 13, 26, 29, 32, 46, 47, 50, 55, 63, 64, 66, 69, 82, 92; Thinstock: 80, 88

*Runner's World* ® is a registered trademark of Rodale Inc.

Text written by Cree Hale Krull.

Printed and bound in the U.K. by CPI Bath using acid-free paper from sustainable resources.

**Library of Congress Catalog-in-Publication data is on file with the publisher.**

ISBN-13 978–1–59486–372–5 paperback
ISBN-10 1–59486–372–1 paperback

**Distributed to the trade by Holtzbrinck Publishers**

2 4 6 8 10 9 7 5 3 1 paperback

⟐ **RODALE**
LIVE YOUR WHOLE LIFE™

We inspire and enable people to improve their lives and the world around them
For more of our products visit **rodalestore.com** or call 800-848-4735

# CONTENTS

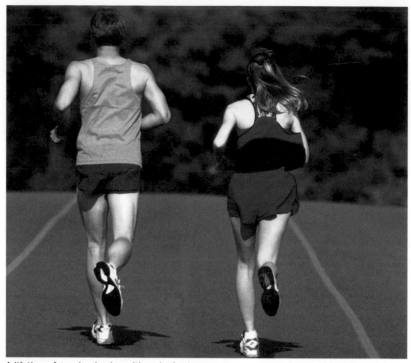

A lifetime of running begins with a single step.

# Introduction

Congratulations—you've just taken the most important step on the rewarding path to becoming a runner: picking up this book to read and learn more about it. Whether you're already running, taking it up again after a layoff, or interested in the sport for the first time, this book contains practical advice, training guidance, injury tips, and information that will help you think of yourself as a runner.

At *Runner's World* magazine, we believe that anyone can run, given the proper motivation and knowledge. To that end, we've organized this book to guide you step-by-step into the subject. In the beginning, it's all about preparation; in the middle, running itself takes center stage, and toward the end, we focus on what lies ahead. Part I, *Why Run?*, for example, deals with your mental preparation, from dispelling the illusions you may have heard about running to understanding its many benefits. Experienced runners will tell you that even though running seems like a purely physical endeavor, it relies on a firm psychological foundation of enthusiasm, commitment, and experience. In other words, if you get your mind running, your feet will follow.

Part II, *Getting Ready*, moves you into physical preparation. "Know thyself," goes the old maxim, and the opening chapters of this section offer advice on preparing to run by checking your current level of physical fitness. What's the only gear you'll need? Running shoes, to be honest, and perhaps an article or two of athletic wear. We bring you up to speed on shoes and clothing, then move on to food—the what, when and how of eating well for optimum running. Lastly, *Getting Ready* takes you through the basics of warming up, cooling down, and stretching, with in-depth descriptions of the best stretches to keep you strong and limber.

## THE RUNNING PLANS

Ready to run? Part III, *The Running Plans*, is the place to go. If you have no prior experience running, check out the 30/30 Plan, which provides a month-long program to get you started. If you have some running experience, the 10-week Run/Walk Plan will build your endurance. And the All-in-One workout will provide the next step in your progress as a runner by challenging your mind, muscles, and lungs. This section also introduces you to the concept and practice of *speed work*—structured workouts that use specific types of running (up hills, for example) to deliver increased stamina and strength. And because injury prevention should always be one of your priorities, we wrap up *The Running Plans* with a primer on how to know when your body is off its mark, and what to do about it.

One of the many joys of running is belonging to a community of runners, and Part IV, *Getting Out* provides valuable tips about different ways to get involved in social running. From finding a running buddy, to joining the group run in your town, to surfing the Web's online running communities, we've got all of the advice you need to get started. There's even a section on one of the newest trends in training runners: coaches who work with you *online*.

## BEYOND THE BASICS

There is always another level to reach for, as you'll learn in Part V, *Next Steps*. Encompassing elements ranging from setting goals, staying motivated, and keeping a training log, to cross-training in complementary sports like cycling and swimming, *Next Steps* includes lots of running know-how. And because no book on running would be complete without a discussion of competition, we end *Getting Started* with tips on how to run your first race.

Use this book as a reference for the basics of running, as inspiration for the days when you need a little motivation, and as a guide for taking your running from where it is to where you want it to be. Every runner, no matter how fast or far they are able to run, started off on Day One with a mixture of enthusiasm, curiosity, and beginner's anxiety. If you're at that moment, or if you've come back to it after some time spent not running, this book is for you—to support your new life as a runner. Everything in this book has been thoroughly researched and is eminently do-able, so read up, lace up, and start running; you have no idea how much fun you'll have until you get started.

## I WISH I HAD KNOWN . . .

At *Runner's World,* we already know what you'll soon find out: 99 percent of runners are friendly, helpful people. That's why we checked in with veteran runners and asked them this: What do you know now that you wish you knew when you started? Whether you're just starting out, or have been running for decades, you'll learn something from their answers, which you'll find scattered throughout the pages of this book. Here's the first:

"I wish I would have been less self-conscious when I started, but I listened to a group of women runners who thought they were on display when they ran. Eventually I saw beyond that. Now I run for me, and I don't care what others think about it."

—Mary, age 45
Years running: 5

# PART I:
# WHY RUN?

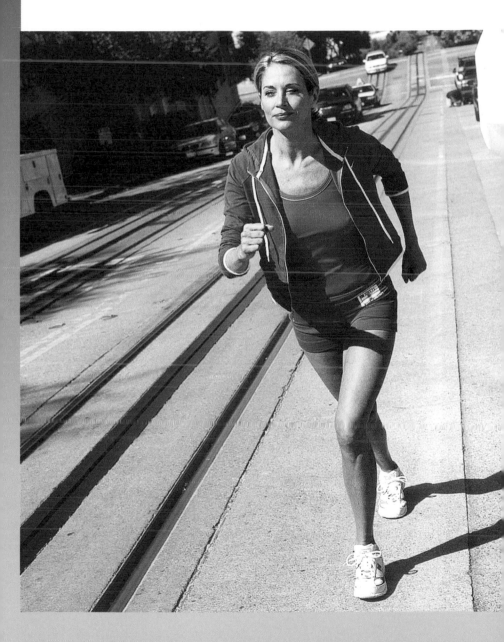

# The Joys of Running

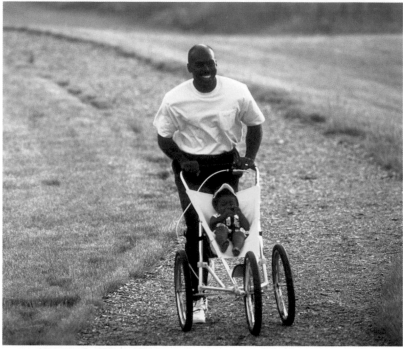

Once you start running, you'll want to share the love.

Running is like love; once you've experienced it, you understand forever what a blissful thing it can be. But just as you might struggle to impart to the lovelorn what it feels like to have found your soul mate, there are aspects of running that you'll really understand only once you've settled into that steady rhythm of footfall and breath.

With that said, here are just some of the tangible benefits you can reap from running.

**It's easy** If you can walk, you can run—any time of the year, anywhere you happen to find yourself. It's just that simple.

**Fits into almost any schedule** It's hard to find a workout that delivers more benefit in just 20 or 30 minutes than running. It's a tremendously efficient activity that gets you fit faster than any other fitness regimen.

**It's uncomplicated** You get out of running what you put into it. In a complex world, running is a refreshingly simple and straightforward activity. The stopwatch and pedometer never lie, so you always know where you stand (or run, as it were). And it doesn't require lots of expensive gear. All you need to get started is a good pair of running shoes (see page 24–27).

**Weight loss** Nothing beats running for sheer calorie-burning power. Thirty minutes of running burns 40 percent more calories than its nearest competitor, cycling.

**Improved muscle tone** Whether you're interested in toning your legs, tightening your midsection, or simply looking as good as you feel, running is a proven means to this end.

**Opportunity for exploration** Ever feel lethargic or disoriented after a long car or plane ride? Join the ranks of runners who routinely explore their new locales with a workout. Not only does running help you get your bearings in a new environment, it helps reset your biological clock if you've crossed time zones, and of course, it gets your body moving again. This is an especially welcome benefit for business people.

**Sets an example for the kids** The active adults of tomorrow need active role models now, and running is a great way to set that example for children. Your road race can easily become a family affair, as many competitions include elements for all ages, such as (very) short distance walk/runs for toddlers and other child-friendly activities after the race.

## ⟩⟩ WHERE SHOULD I RUN?

You can run almost anywhere, as long as it's safe, and you enjoy it. The best running routes are scenic, well lit, free of traffic, and well populated. Think of running as a way to explore new territory. Use your watch to gauge your distance, and set out on a new adventure on each run. Ask other runners about the best local routes. If you don't yet know other runners, try the Internet. Good search terms include your town or neighborhood name and the words "running" and "routes."

**Better sleep** As long as you end your runs at least 3 hours before you want to go to sleep, you'll find that consistent running delivers restful hours like you haven't experienced in years. Not surprisingly, the more vigorously you work out, the deeper you'll sleep later on.

**Increased fitness for other sports** So maybe running isn't at the center of your athletic dreams. No matter—the increased stamina and core fitness you get from running can benefit you in almost any athletic endeavor. Call it the universal cross-training exercise.

**Increased brain power** Some studies suggest running improves a variety of mental functions. One study recently conducted in Japan found that a 12-week running program significantly improved the reaction times and memory performance of participants.

Other studies point to running's pronounced beneficial effect on the hippocampus—the part of the brain that converts short-term memories to long-term ones. The bottom line: Running is good for your brain.

**It feels good** There's an old adage about running: It feels good only once it's over. Whether you find yourself enjoying running in the moment or not (and many people do), you will, without fail, feel better after you run, and that good feeling can stay with you for hours,

## PSYCH YOURSELF UP

Need that little something extra to get started on your running journey? Develop your own runner's ritual for building up your enthusiasm. The routine you build now will also come in handy later on, on those off days when you can't possibly imagine lacing up your shoes.

- Sit down with a glass of water an hour or two before your run, and visualize yourself performing your workout with ease.
- Listen to some energetic music before and even while you run (small lightweight MP3 players are a major improvement over portable cassette or CD players in this regard).
- Stoke your enthusiasm for running with an inspiring book, magazine article, or even a film about athletic achievement.

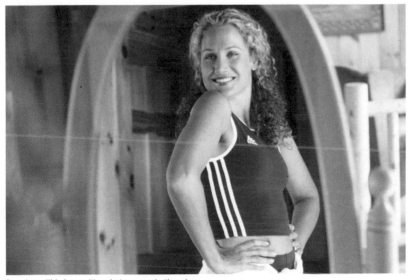

Running will help you like what you see in the mirror.

making running the ultimate pick-me-up after a day's work. Research has even found that running (and exercise in general) reduces anxiety and even depression.

**Increased energy** Non-runners often don't understand how one can actually feel more energetic after a run. The exact cause of this energy windfall remains elusive, but studies have demonstrated a connection between high-exertion activities like running and subsequent feelings of productivity, and well-being. Go for a run and skip the coffee—you won't miss it. Go to a road race and take a look at the well-toned masters runners (usually runners over 40). Their youthful looks belie their age.

**Heightened creativity** Running is more than just the stress release. Writers, artists, musicians, software engineers, and many others use running to work through creative blocks and to make decisions with increased clarity. Get that body and mind working in concert with a good run.

**Enhanced self-discipline** Studies show that the most successful people are those with a modicum of talent and an enormous amount of self-discipline. Like your hamstrings and quadriceps, self-discipline is a muscle you develop over the course of a running program. So start running, and see the benefits play out in all aspects of your life.

# Running Myths

Most of what you may have heard about running is wrong: It won't wreck your knees and it isn't only for skinny people. It doesn't have to be boring and it won't make your uterus drop (if you're a woman). We've all heard reasons why "running is bad for you," but the fact is that people who make those arguments are usually ill-informed. On the next few pages, we set the record straight on some of the most common inaccuracies about the simplest and perhaps oldest athletic activity on earth.

### RUNNING IS BAD FOR YOUR KNEES

Let's start with the most persistent falsehood. The knee joint has been fine-tuned by millennia of evolution to withstand running; and some evolutionary physiologists even claim that for humans, running, not walking, is the most natural form of movement. By toning the body in multiple ways, running can actually strengthen joints. Just talk to U.S. ultramarathoner Dean Karnazes, who competes in running events much longer than the 26.2 mile (42.2 km) marathon. His quest to become the first person to run 300 miles (483 km) without stopping should certainly qualify him to address the issue of wear and tear on the joints. His knees, according to his doctor, are in great shape.

### RUNNING IS BAD FOR YOUR HEART

Make no mistake—running is cardiovascular exercise par excellence, and studies show that engaging in regular exercise like running can extend your life anywhere from 2 to 9 years. Knowing the state of your cardiovascular fitness before you begin a running program–whether you're just starting out or returning to the sport—is essential, and will equip you with the confidence to push yourself when the time is right.

### ONLY THIN PEOPLE SHOULD RUN

People of all body types run regularly and even start and finish races of all lengths. You don't have to have the perfect body to begin a running program. Start running,

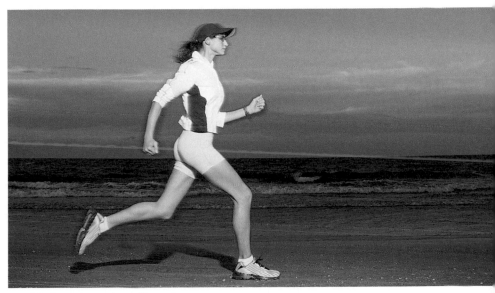

Actually, running can be *good* for your knees.

and your inner athlete will start to show, regardless of how large, small, thin, or stout you are. Running can reshape not only your body, but your life as well.

## RUNNING IS ONLY FOR THE YOUNG

The old adage, "if you can walk, you can run," holds true at nearly any age. In fact, many runners come to the sport in adulthood, without prior experience in high school or college athletics. Is running for the young, or do runners simply look younger? The benefits you see in your face alone after running a few weeks may convince you of the latter.

## YOU NEED LOTS OF STAMINA TO RUN

Running *builds* stamina; and if you begin and train wisely—increasing the amount of time you run slowly and taking enough rest days—you'll have all the endurance you need to run.

## RUNNING IS BORING AND LONELY

The truth is that running is more social than it has ever been before—a sport engaged in by formal running clubs and informal running groups of spouses, friends, and co-workers. Its very pervasiveness means you probably already know someone who runs, and with that connection, your network of running buddies begins. No one need be a lonely runner anymore.

## JOGGERS AREN'T REAL RUNNERS

If you take only one thing from this book let it be this: All runners walk, and all runners jog (that is, run slowly). Take heart knowing that you and Olympic marathoners the world over walk and run slowly from time to time because it is the right thing at a given point in their training. As an athlete, you can and should work out in the best possible way for increased stamina and achievement; running, walking, and jogging are all aspects of your workout, and none should carry a stigma of weakness or non-athleticism.

## YOU NEED PERFECT STRIDE

It may surprise you to know that even the most frequently heard tip regarding stride—run "tall" with an erect posture—is not beyond debate in the running community, and though we stand behind the stride guidelines offered in this book, your growth as a runner will bring you in touch with many different schools of practice. Put simply, your perfect stride reflects your unique physiology, and like most things, evolves over time, as you get deeper into the sport.

## WOMEN SHOULDN'T RUN

This is an old one, but it still crops up from time to time. Once upon a time, the rumor started that if a woman ran, she risked having her uterus drop (not true). Then the argument evolved into "women

## ⟫ GOING BEYOND HER LIMITS

When your left leg is amputated at the age of 7, no one expects you to run at age 11, much less compete in seven triathlons before the age of 30. But low expectations haven't stopped Sarah Reinertsen of Solana Beach, California, from competing in the Hawaii Ironman Triathlon—the first woman with a prosthetic leg to do so—and winning the female leg-amputee division of the International Triathlon World Championships in New Zealand. Reinertsen continues to compete and show the world what hard work, dedication, and a no-limits attitude can accomplish.

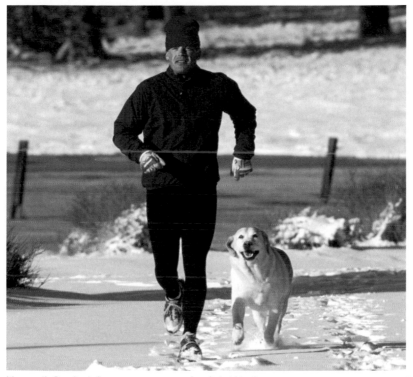

It's no myth: Running is for everyone—even your four-footed friends.

shouldn't run long distances." This one probably started after the 1928 Olympics. Back then, the longest race in which women could officially compete was the 800-yard run. That year, the race was held on a hot and humid evening; afterward, several of the women collapsed on the track. Despite a new world record being set by Germany's Lina Radke, the Olympic committee saw fit to restrict the longest race for women to 220 yards—that rule stayed on the books until 1960. It wasn't until 1984 that women's marathoning became an official Olympic event.

Women can, do, and should run—if that's what they want to do. Although men are faster than women at most distances, it's interesting to note that in recent years, women have beaten men in the 50- and 100-mile distances. Of course, it doesn't have to be a competition or a war between the sexes. The point is that men *and* women can reap the benefits of running while enjoying it.

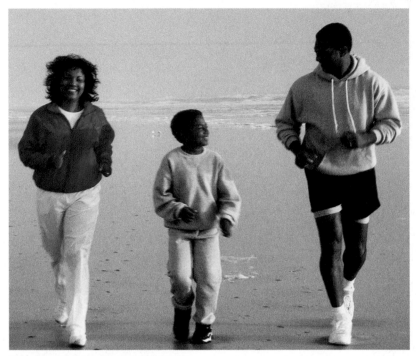

Make running a family affair and get fit together.

## IGNORE THE MYTHS: YOU CAN BE A RUNNER

If you have any doubts about whether running is for you, here's some advice: Deep down, the most important reason to be a runner is very simple—you want to be one. Always remember that your body knows how to run. You're a primate with a predator's genes, and although a 20-minute run through the park is unlikely to engage that inborn ability to run like hell from a saber-toothed tiger, it's comforting, even inspiring, to know you're so equipped. Running puts you in touch with something fundamental about the human experience, and you're as uniquely qualified to partake of it as anyone else.

The runner you become starts with your intention. Whether you prefer running alone or with friends, for the thrill of competition or because it makes you feel good about yourself, it all starts within you. Hold onto the image of yourself as a runner, and remind yourself that you are as much a runner as anyone else on this planet. With this in mind, it won't be long until you believe it.

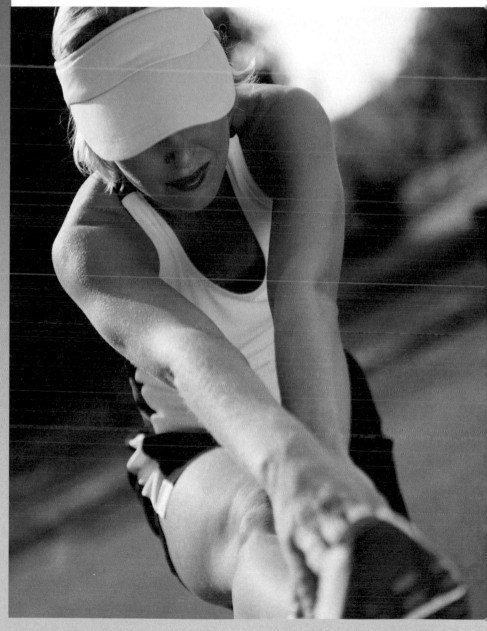

# PART II:
# GETTING READY

# What's Your Starting Point?

**Before you start the running programs in this book, it's a smart idea to determine your current fitness level. That way, not only do you begin with more realistic expectations, but when you finish the programs, you can redo these tests and have hard numbers telling you how much you've improved over the course of your training.**

The way you're going to ascertain your current fitness is by performing The 1.5-Mile Field Test, developed by the Cooper Institute, a nonprofit research organization located in Dallas, Texas, that studies health and fitness. This test measures your cardiovascular fitness, which is a good indicator of overall health. More specifically, it calculates your VO2 *max*, a number that indicates how efficiently your cardiovascular system moves blood to your muscles while you're working out, and how well your muscles use that oxygen.

## THE FIELD TEST

For the test itself, walk, run, or run and walk a distance of 1.5 miles– that's six times around a standard athletics track. The goal is to finish that distance in as little time as

## CALCULATE YOUR VO2 MAX

Here's the formula to calculate your VO2 max: In this example, we'll use a 160-pound man.

VO2 max = 88.02 − .1656 x (body weight in kg[a]) − 2.76 x (time in minutes it took you to complete the distance[b]) + 3.716 x (gender[c])

  a: Body weight in kilograms: Divide your weight in pounds by 2.2. For a 160-pound man:
  $$160 \div 2.2 = 72.72 \text{ kg}$$

  b: Time in minutes: Convert seconds to minutes by dividing the seconds by 60.
  For example: a 1.5 mile running time of 12 minutes, 30 seconds would be converted to 12.5. (30 ÷ 60 = .5 minute)

  c: Use 1 for male and 0 for female
  VO2 max = 88.02 - [.1656 x 72.72 kg] - [2.76 x 15.47 + 3.716] x 1
  VO2 max = 88.02 - [12.04] - [46.41] x 1
  VO2 max = 88.02 - 12.04 - 46.41 x 1 = 29.57

possible without exhausting yourself. Once you have finished, record your time in minutes and seconds.

For the next step, there is some math to do, but it's simple if you break it down into steps (See *Calculate Your VO2 Max*, opposite).

Once you know your VO2 max, compare it to the numbers in the tables below, then stash it away for the next 3½ months. If your initial VO2 is below average, don't be disheartened: Running will certainly improve it.

## MEN

| Percentile | 20–29 | 30–39 | 40–49 | 50–59 | 60+ |
|---|---|---|---|---|---|
| 90 | 51.4 | 50.4 | 48.2 | 45.3 | 42.5 |
| 80 | 48.2 | 46.8 | 44.1 | 41.0 | 38.1 |
| 70 | 46.8 | 44.6 | 41.8 | 38.5 | 35.3 |
| 60 | 44.2 | 42.4 | 39.9 | 36.7 | 33.6 |
| 50 | 42.5 | 41.0 | 38.1 | 35.2 | 31.8 |
| 40 | 41.0 | 38.9 | 36.7 | 33.8 | 30.2 |
| 30 | 39.5 | 37.4 | 35.1 | 32.3 | 28.7 |
| 20 | 37.1 | 35.4 | 33.0 | 30.2 | 26.5 |
| 10 | 34.5 | 32.5 | 30.9 | 28.0 | 23.1 |

*Age* (column header spanning 20–29 through 60+)

## WOMEN

| Percentile | 20–29 | 30–39 | 40–49 | 50–59 | 60+ |
|---|---|---|---|---|---|
| 90 | 44.2 | 41.0 | 39.5 | 35.2 | 35.2 |
| 80 | 41.0 | 38.6 | 36.3 | 32.3 | 31.2 |
| 70 | 38.1 | 36.7 | 33.8 | 30.9 | 29.4 |
| 60 | 36.7 | 34.6 | 32.3 | 29.4 | 27.2 |
| 50 | 35.2 | 33.8 | 30.9 | 28.2 | 25.8 |
| 40 | 33.8 | 32.3 | 29.5 | 26.9 | 24.5 |
| 30 | 32.3 | 30.5 | 28.3 | 25.5 | 23.8 |
| 20 | 30.6 | 28.7 | 26.5 | 24.3 | 22.8 |
| 10 | 28.4 | 26.5 | 25.1 | 22.3 | 20.8 |

*Age* (column header spanning 20–29 through 60+)

90 or above: Well above average
70 to 89: Above average
50 to 69: Average
30 to 49: Below average
29 and below: Well below average

*Source: The Physical Fitness Specialist Certification Manual, The Cooper Institute, Dallas, TX, reprinted with permission.*

# Time for a Checkup?

As good for you as running is, it's still a vigorous, and at times strenuous, form of exercise. That means if you're over age 40 or simply haven't been to the doctor in several years, it's important to have a full physical exam before beginning any of the running programs in this book.

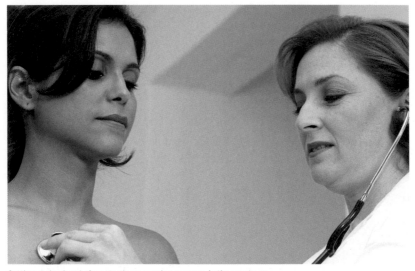

Getting a checkup before starting a running program is the way to go.

A regular physical is useful not only as a preventative measure, but what you learn from your checkup can also serve as a benchmark against which to measure your progress in the months and years to come.

## WHAT'S UP AT THE DOC'S

Has it been a few years (or more) since your last physical? No problem. Talk to your health care provider about your plans to begin running, and let him or her know

that you're interested in having the following tests performed in order to evaluate your starting point.

**Blood pressure and heart rate** These is basic information you'll get from a physical. Ideally, your blood pressure should be below 120/80. The average adult's resting heart rate (or RHR) is around 72 beats per minute (or BPM).

**Exercise stress test** Also known as a submax test, it is performed to make sure you have

# WATCH YOUR HEART RATE

Your resting heart rate is one number you'll want to keep an eye on as you progress in your running program. As you become more fit, your RHR will begin to fall. That's because your heart is getting stronger and can pump more blood with each beat.

After running for several months, your average RHR may drop to 60 or below. The RHR of elite athletes can be much lower—seven-time Tour de France winner Lance Armstrong's RHR is 32 BPM. Many runners record their RHR every morning in their running logs as a way to gauge the effectiveness of their training and to make sure they're not training too hard. An increased RHR may indicate illness coming on or overtraining.

To measure your RHR, simply place the first two fingertips of one hand on the inside of the other wrist, below the thumb, and count the number of times your heart beats in 1 minute. Do this first thing in the morning, before you even get out of bed, for the most accurate results.

no cardiovascular issues that may surface when you exercise. During the test, you'll walk or run on a treadmill while monitors record your heart and lung function. Keep in mind that if you're younger than 40 or have no other pertinent risk factors, your doctor may feel that this test is unnecessary.

**The sound of your heart** Your doctor will use a stethoscope to listen for arrhythmias (irregular heart beats) and heart murmurs, which are caused by leaky heart valves.

**Blood tests** Maintaining healthy levels of blood cholesterol, triglycerides, and blood glucose is important, as your training could aggravate an undiagnosed condition. Your HDL (so-called "good") cholesterol levels should be above 50 mg/dL (1.293 mmol/L). The LDL ("bad") levels should be below 100 mg/dL (2.586 mmol/L). Triglycerides (the building blocks of fats in your blood) should be lower than 150 mg/dL (1.6935 mmol/L), and blood glucose readings below 100 mg/dL (5.56 mmol/L).

Make sure that your doctor reviews all of the test results with you and, if you are unclear about any of your results, don't hesitate to ask him or her for further explanation.

# Gearing Up

When compared to other sports–skiing, cycling, golfing–
running is the least gear intensive. But there is one vital
piece of gear: the running shoe. Wearing the wrong shoe
can lead to problems ranging from blisters to stress frac-
tures. That's why we begin this section with detailed advice
about choosing the right shoe. From there, we discuss the
clothing you'll need to run comfortably when it's hot and
dry, wet and rainy, or cold and snowy.

## CHOOSE THE RIGHT RUNNING SHOES

Choosing the proper running shoe isn't quite as complicated as nuclear fission, but for a beginner it can be daunting to sort through all the models and high-tech shoe systems. The best place to start the shoe selection process is at a running shoe store.

A running store should be a fun place to go and shop. But with all the new, colorful models on the shoe wall and the slim, fit people gathered about, it can also be an intimidating place for a newcomer. Still, a good running store should cater to the needs of the beginner as well as the experienced. If you don't feel the store's salespeople are receptive to your needs, talk over your head, or are condescending, go someplace else. Before you head to the store, it's a good idea to have a basic understanding of how your feet work and learn about the basic varieties of shoes avail-able — it'll help you make a more informed purchase.

## HOW YOUR FOOT MOVES

Once you start running and shop-ping for shoes, you'll begin to hear the word *pronation* a lot. It refers to a natural biomechanical process: When your foot comes down and strikes the ground, the first part to make contact with the ground is the outside edge of your heel. As your foot rolls forward, it also rolls slightly inward, so that the ball of your foot behind your first and second toes takes more of the impact than the rest of your forefoot. Lastly, as your heel leaves the ground to begin the next stride, the ball of your foot pushes your entire foot forward. In a nutshell, that's pronation.

There are two variations on pronation. The first, *overpronation*, is common to people with flat feet or low arches. It involves a greater amount of inward roll toward the ball of the foot. Overpronation (when not kept in check by the right shoes) commonly causes injuries to the knees and lower legs.

The second variation on pronation occurs when your foot doesn't roll inward enough on each stride. This is called *supination* (also called underpronation). It can result in its own injuries if left uncorrected, since the leg and hips are absorbing the impact of heel strike without the assistance of a good pronating roll.

## CHOOSING A SHOE

The best place to start is by taking the Wet Test (see page 26). Take time to do it now and make note of the results. Your foot shape and degree of pronation determine the kind of running shoe you need. Luckily, most running shoes will give you a clear indication of their characteristics just by the shape of their sole. In general, the soles of running shoes come in

## THE PERFECT PAIR

First of all, a well-sized running shoe will be snug, but not tight. Make sure you can press the end of your thumb between the end of your longest toe and the front end of the shoe's toe box (the area covering your toes). First-time buyers routinely buy running shoes too small for their feet, and find their toes cramped as their workouts progress. Your heel should be held firmly in place without pain or slippage when you run. Similarly, the upper part of the shoe should grip the top of your foot snugly yet comfortably, without irritation, or too light a touch. Comfort and fit are the key elements to strive for when choosing your shoe, so don't compromise on either. There's always another shoe to try on.

## TAKE THE WET TEST

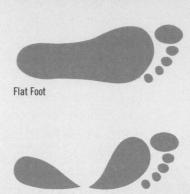

Flat Foot

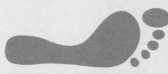

High Arch

Normal

Our "Wet Test" is a quick and easy way of discovering your degree of pronation. Lay a piece of brown craft paper (or take apart a brown paper bag) on a hard floor (no carpeting). Lightly wet the sole of your foot with some water, and then make a footprint on the paper. Pay close attention to the wet areas on the paper.

A flat foot will show up as a complete imprint of your sole. Specifically, the arch of your foot will be wet and make direct contact with the paper. This footprint means that you probably have a tendency to overpronate.

A high-arched foot will dampen the paper with an imprint of the heel, ball, and toes of your sole, with marginal wetting along the outside edge and no imprint at all of your arch on the paper. More than likely, this imprint means you have a tendency to supinate.

A normal foot imprint will look similar to the high-arched imprint, but will show a strong outline along the outer edge of the foot connecting the heel imprint to the imprint of the ball of the foot. This imprint means you are probably a normal pronator.

three shapes—straight, or flat; semi-curved; and curved–which correspond roughly to the three types of footprints revealed by the Wet Test. If you have a flat foot, low-to-no arch, and/or are an overpronator, choose a shoe with a straight sole. If you have a high arch and/or are a supinator, choose a shoe with a curved sole. Finally, if you have a normal arch and/or are a normal pronator, choose a shoe with a semi-curved sole.

There are other variables to consider besides a shoe's sole shape. For instance, motion control shoes are designed specifically for overpronators. The three characteristics common to motion-control shoes are: (1) a thick, firm mid-sole (constructed of one or two materials, the so-called "dual density" mid-sole); (2) straight sole for maximum foot support; and (3) a firm and snug heel "counter," contoured molding that stretches around your heel, to control rear-foot movement.

Cushioned shoes, designed for supinators, promote the natural rolling action of your foot, rather than control it. A soft, cushioned mid-sole is paired with a curved or semi-curved sole to give your foot the flexibility it needs to roll properly from heel to toe.

For those lucky runners with normal pronation, shoe companies offer a multitude of options that run the gamut. Stability or neutral-cushioning are adjectives frequently used in the running world to describe shoes for the normal pronator.

## DRESS FOR THE WEATHER

Wouldn't it be nice if your workout always took place under sunny skies, with low humidity and a fresh breeze at your back? Alas, there will be days when you are faced with almost every other kind of weather. How should you prepare? Glad you asked.

**Cold weather basics** Strive to be "comfortably cool." Your body heats up as you run, so feeling a bit chilly as you begin your workout is not necessarily a bad sign. Keep your layers thin, and without breaking your budget, consider investing in a synthetic first layer, which will pull (or "wick") sweat away from your skin. Avoid cotton clothing at all costs in cold, or cold and wet weather. When wet, cotton actually pulls your body heat away from you.

In most climates, you can get by all winter with just three thin layers for your torso: a moisture-wicking first layer against your skin; a thin fleece, wool or acrylic sweater for warmth; and an outer jacket (a "shell") of nylon, or similar wind-breaking fabric, preferably with a hood to protect your neck, ears, and scalp.

For your legs, synthetic or synthetic- and wool-blend running tights are a good investment, offering warmth and support for your muscles. When it comes to your feet, remember that not all socks are created equal. Wool and

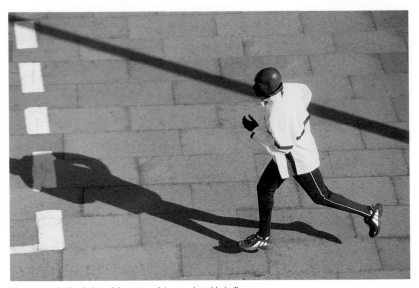

Wearing synthetics helps wick away moisture and avoid chafing.

synthetic-wool blends will reward you with warmer feet in cold weather than cotton, but bear in mind that wearing your thickest pair of wool socks could be a prescription for blisters if you shopped for shoes wearing thin socks.

As for hats, gloves, and so on, you probably already have what you need in your closet—as long as it's not cotton.

**Wet weather basics** For those rainy days that are too cold for comfort, keep your shell handy. Gore-Tex™ will keep you dry while allowing your perspiration to evaporate.

Caring for your extremities is just as important in wet weather as in cold. Wear a brimmed hat or cap to shield your eyes from the rain, and wear gloves if it's cold. As for your socks and shoes, they're likely to get wet, so prepare yourself for a day or two of air-drying your shoes once you're back inside. To facilitate the drying process, stuff your shoes with crumpled up newspaper, changing it as it absorbs the water.

**Hot weather basics** Protecting yourself from excessive heat and humidity is paramount in hot weather, so keep in mind the usefulness of a hat or visor to shield your head and/or face. In addition, don't forget to stay well hydrated. Because the incidence of skin cancer is increasing all around the world, shielding your skin from the harsh rays of the sun is vital year-round—not just in summertime. Wear sunglasses with UV protection, and heed these other rules of thumb, which are especially important for runners who spend long periods of time outdoors and in the sun:

Avoid running during the sun's peak hours (generally 10 A.M. to 4 P.M.).

Always wear a broad-spectrum sunscreen with a sun protection factor (SPF) of 15 or higher.

Reapply sunscreen often, especially to your ears, nose, and lips, the parts of your body that are more susceptible to sun damage.

The sun's ultraviolet rays can penetrate many types of clothing, so if you're especially fair-skinned, you may want to consider purchasing special UV-blocking apparel.

During any physical exams, tell your doctor that you spend lots of time outdoors so that he or she will be sure to check your skin for signs of skin cancer.

## THE SPORTS BRA

For women runners, having the right running bra can mean the difference between having an enjoyable experience and one you'd rather forget. There are three types of sports bras on today's market: those that compress the breasts, those that encapsulate them, and others, called combination bras, which do a little of both. Compression-style bras use the pressure of the fabric

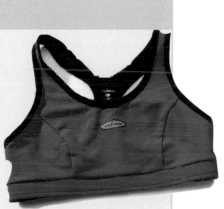

to squeeze or press the breasts flat against the chest, limiting movement. This style is favored by small- to medium-breasted women. An encapsulation style bra limits movement by surrounding and supporting the breasts with reinforced seams or wire (like an underwire bra); this type is preferred by larger breasted women. Not surprisingly, the combination style "combines" compression and encapsulation, and is popular with both medium- and large-breasted women. With so many options for sports bras, comfort should ultimately dictate your choice.

# Eat and Drink Right

Running offers great rewards, mentally, physically, and emotionally. What it can do for your metabolism is nothing short of amazing. Strong running places enormous caloric demands on your body even as it ramps up your metabolism. If that sounds like a great prescription for losing weight, it is, but remember the old saying, "garbage in, garbage out." What, when, and how you eat are important components to your success as a runner; in that vein, we offer these simple guidelines.

## THE BEST FOODS FOR RUNNERS

Runners, like everyone else, should emphasize good nutrition right down to the fundamental building blocks. It's not just about eating any old proteins, carbohydrates, and fat, after all—it's about eating the right ones. The dynamite foods that follow will get you going with the right nutrition, right now. Presented here are more than twenty staples for your kitchen, organized by food category.

## GRAINS

**Brown rice** There are several varieties to choose from, ranging from short-grain to fragrant long-grain basmati, so you're bound to find one that suits your preferences. All offer unparalleled nutritional value when it comes to complex carbohydrates, fiber, vitamins, and minerals. When combined with beans, brown rice creates a complete protein that can replace animal sources like meat or dairy products in your diet.

**Buckwheat pasta** Also known as soba noodles, buckwheat pasta offers more whole grains and is higher in minerals and carbohydrates than regular pasta. Add them to soup, or use in a stir-fry.

**Oatmeal** A serving of oats provides plenty of slow-release carbohydrates, which gives you more sustained energy than refined carbohydrates, such as white flour or sugar. Oatmeal has also been shown to lower cholesterol. Have it anytime, and add skim milk and dried fruit for extra nutritional punch. Instant

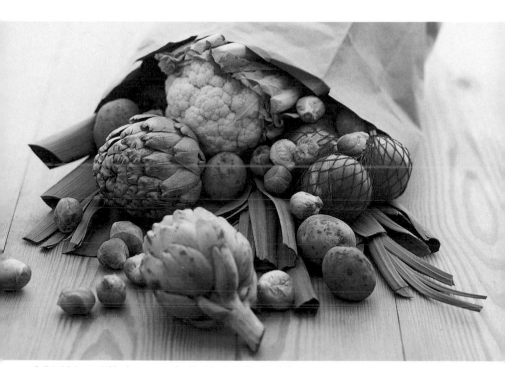

A diet rich in vegetables lowers many health risks, including heart disease.

oatmeal offers much the same benefits as rolled oats, but avoid presweetened varieties, which have a high sugar content.

**Whole-grain bread** Breads made with complete flours like whole wheat, rye, and spelt contain more fiber and nutrients than breads made with lighter, whiter flours. So when you reach for bread, go for rustic varieties like wheat-rye peasant loaves, whole-grain sourdoughs, and multigrain sandwich bread, and hold off on the baguettes and brioche which are filled with empty calories.

## VEGETABLES AND LEGUMES

**Asparagus** A good source of vitamins A and C, asparagus can be eaten raw, but it's best steamed or sautéed. Asparagus also provides potassium, an important electrolyte mineral that helps the body maintain fluid levels and regulate blood pressure. Runners lose potassium through perspiration, so they need to replenish it after a good workout.

**Beans** These are among the most versatile and nutrition-packed foods in the vegetable kingdom. Varieties such as pinto, lentil, gar-

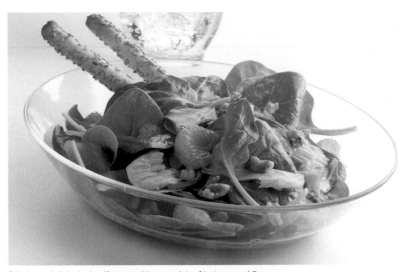

Salads needn't be boring if you combine a variety of textures and flavors.

banzo, and green peas are rich in protein, fiber, and iron, and they're low in fat. They're a classic ingredient in soups and stews, tossed in salads, or served with brown rice for a complete carb-protein meal.

**Dark Leafy Greens** Think collards, kale, chard, and spinach—the darker the better. Leafy greens are excellent sautéed with garlic and olive oil, and will boost your intake of vitamins A and C, plus fiber and iron. And don't neglect lettuce, but choose the dark varieties like Romaine or red-leaf rather than pale, nutrition-free iceberg.

## FRUIT

**Bananas** Versatile, convenient, and delicious, bananas are packed with carbohydrates and potassium.

**Cantaloupe** Half a melon provides a day's worth of vitamins A and C. Melons are rich in beta-carotene, an antioxidant vitamin that can help prevent both cancer and heart disease. Great as a post-run snack or with cottage cheese for a light and tasty lunch.

**Oranges** One orange provides all the vitamin C you need in a day, so you'll be well-fortified against upper-respiratory infections that are common during periods of intense training. Plus, vitamin C's antioxidants will protect you from muscle damage and soreness.

## DAIRY

**Low-fat cheese** Versatile choices such as provolone, mozzarella, and feta are excellent for salads, sandwiches, and pizzas, and provide calcium (especially important for women) and protein.

**Low-fat or non-fat yogurt** Any kind, plain or with fruit, provides calcium, protein, and plenty of energizing carbohydrates, making it an excellent grab-and-go food.

**Skim milk** This nonfat alternative to whole milk comes loaded with protein, carbohydrates, calcium, and potassium. What's more, protein from milk is absorbed particularly well.

## SEAFOOD

**Mackerel** This fish is high in protein as well as omega-3 fatty acids, which contribute to healthy cell membranes, proper brain functioning, and reduced risk for heart disease. Stick with fresh or canned mackerel as opposed to smoked, since the smoking process reduces the omega-3 content dramatically.

**Salmon** Exceptionally high in protein and omega-3 fatty acids, salmon can be prepared in dozens of ways. Even canned salmon is great for you.

**Tuna** High in protein and omega-3s, tuna is convenient and economical. Toss it in pita bread with lettuce and tomato for an excellent sandwich.

## MEAT AND POULTRY

**Chicken and turkey** For lean protein, eat chicken and turkey baked, grilled, or broiled (remove the skin before eating). Keep sliced turkey on hand for quick protein snacks and easy-to-make lunches.

**Lamb** There's lots of protein, iron, and zinc (which aids in muscle repair and sexual function) in a lamb roast. Make sure to trim the fat after cooking.

**Lean roast beef** With an abundance of vitamin B, iron, and zinc, lean roast beef is the most nutrient-dense red meat.

## PROTEIN ALTERNATIVES

**Nuts** They contain heart-healthy fat and lots of minerals, so eat a variety of nuts (or nut butter) several times a week. Add them to dried fruit, such as cranberries, for a tasty and healthy trail mix.

**Soymilk** Often fortified with calcium and vitamin E, soymilk is an excellent protein source, plus it contains disease-fighting phytochemicals. Soymilk is a great alternative for those who are lactose intolerant.

**Tofu** Made of soybean curd, tofu supplies all the health benefits of soymilk. It's tasty in stir-fries, or crumbled into salads.

## WHEN SHOULD YOU EAT?

To keep their appetites from raging out of control and leading them to make poor food choices, many runners have adopted a "six-meals-a-day" system. That doesn't mean six full-sized meals. Instead of a big lunch at noon, eat half at 10:00 A.M. and the other half at 2:00 P.M., and so on. It will take some practice on your part to find the right times and portions for your individual needs, but with a little practice, you'll master the habit. Adherents of the six-meals-a-day approach report more constant energy throughout the day, without post-meal or mid-afternoon

## SAMPLE SIX-MEAL SCHEDULE

Here's how to break up three square meals into six mini-meals, for a grand total of 2,200 calories:

**Breakfast**

1 packet instant oatmeal with skim milk; 6 ounces calcium-fortified, extra-pulp orange juice

**Morning Snack**

8 ounces fruit yogurt shake

**Lunch**

3 ounces turkey, 1.5 ounces cheese with low-fat mayo, shredded lettuce, and tomato in a whole-wheat wrap; 1 green apple

**Afternoon Snack**

1 whole-wheat bagel or
2 rice cakes with
1 tablespoon peanutbutter

**Dinner**

3 ounces herb-crusted salmon fillet, 1 large mixed green salad with low-fat dressing; 1 cup couscous; 1 cup sautéed broccoli

**Late-night Snack**

1/3 cup granola, 1/2 cup low-fat milk or yogurt, 1/2 cup blueberries or strawberries

Wait at least an hour before running after eating a large meal, or one with relatively higher amounts of protein and fat than carbohydrates (such as, the salmon fillet dinner noted above).

For smaller, quick meals like the afternoon snack of a bagel with peanut butter, you need wait only about twenty minutes before running.

Don't run if more than 3 hours have passed since your last meal—you need energy, so wait a bit and then start your run.

slumps. We've provided a day's menu—see *Sample Six-Meal Schedule*, opposite.

## WATER, WATER EVERYWHERE

The era of drinking "eight 8-ounce glasses of water daily" is over. A better approach is to drink water throughout the day in small amounts until your urine runs clear—this is the most important point. When your urine runs clear, you're well hydrated. If you start out well hydrated, water is the best beverage for runs under an hour.

For runs longer than an hour, or on hot days, try a sports drink. Your thirst will be quenched and

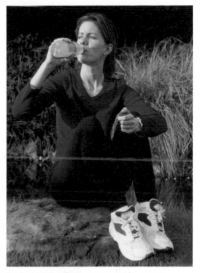
Don't drink too little – or too much – water.

you'll get an easily assimilated dose of carbs and electrolytes (salts your body needs) to keep you running at high efficiency.

## ⟩⟩ HYPONATREMIA

As the ranks of marathoners have swelled in recent years, more average runners are on the road for long periods of time. Although fear of dehydration has dogged endurance athletes for years, the abundance of water—during races, but also during training—has led to a growing number of cases of HYPONATREMIA. This condition occurs when you take in so much water and sweat so much that the sodium levels in your blood drop and your blood thins. Disorientation and weakness result, and in extreme cases, it can lead to brain seizures and death.

Hyponatremia is most likely to strike at the end of a long run on a hot day. Avoid hyponatremia with these simple guidelines: Don't avoid salt in your diet, especially before competitions. Drink sports drinks, rather than water, before, during, and after long runs. And don't ignore dizziness or other signs of the condition.

# Before and After

Any car mechanic will tell you to warm up your engine with an easy idle before driving anywhere. The body's engine works the same way. Yet we're often too rushed to warm up properly. We lace up our shoes and go, heedless of the consequences. That can be a real mistake, since a rushed start makes it difficult to reach the effortless zone of relaxed running we all strive for.

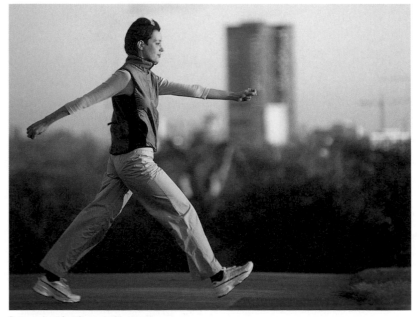

Put your best foot forward with a good warm-up.

The key to a good warm-up is to gradually increase your heart rate and core temperature, while simultaneously pumping blood to your muscles. Skip the warm-up and your body enters mild oxygen debt, which leads to strained muscle fibers and sore legs.

Ensuring a gentle transition from a resting state to vigorous exertion is your warm-up goal every time you run. A proper warm-up leaves you feeling strong and comfortable by mid-run, and it also reduces the risk of injury. If you're tempted to do a little

## MUSCLE PHYSICS

According to the basic laws of physics, muscles will work more efficiently when they are longer, and stretching aids this process; they can exert more force with less effort. This also means that longer muscles are less prone to injury. Consider these simple facts:

- When you first get up in the morning, your muscles and soft tissues are tight. In fact, at that time your muscles are generally about 10 percent shorter than their normal resting length.
- When you start exercising, your muscles stretch up to 10 percent longer than they were before you began. This means you have a 20 percent change in muscle length from the time you get out of bed until your muscles are well warmed up.

pre-run stretching and call that your warm-up, don't. However beneficial stretching is (more on that in the next few pages), it generally doesn't elevate your heart rate or make you perspire, which is what you need to run efficiently. Begin your warm-up by walking or running very slowly to ease your body into the session.

Try these sample warm-ups to reap the maximum benefits from your running:

**Warm-up 1** Walk for 3 minutes to get the blood moving into your muscles. Then alternate 30 to 60 seconds of slow jogging with the same amount of walking for a total of 5 minutes. You should then be ready to ease into your natural training pace.

**Warm-up 2** Gradually increase your walking pace over 5 minutes before you break into a run. This may sound simple, but it requires some effort to pace yourself correctly. Don't count this time as part of your workout itself—you're working up to that.

**Warm-up 3** Walk for 1 to 2 minutes, then shift into a shuffling jog. Your feet should barely clear the ground at first. Gradually start lifting your knees higher and lengthening your stride over the next 10 to 15 minutes; at the end of this period, you can start your workout in earnest. Keep in mind that on morning runs, your body is still waking up and may take a bit longer to reach the warm, relaxed state you're aiming for.

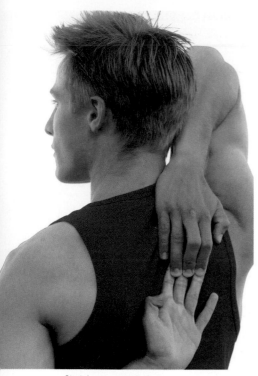

Stretch your upper body, too.

## COOL DOWN...

It can be hard to believe that something as simple as cooling down after your run has such a complex and powerful effect on your physiology. Like closing a book and putting it back on the shelf so you can retrieve it easily the next time you want to read it, cooling down properly starts the process of post-workout recovery. Your muscles will ache less and heal faster, and their performance will improve more quickly when you take a few minutes to bring

your body back to a resting state after exertion. Along with your warm-up, a cool-down should be a staple of your workouts.

Just as your body can be shocked by a sudden increase in activity, it can be unpleasantly surprised when you abruptly stop running. The blood that was pumped quickly back up to your heart by your leg muscles while you ran, will pool in your legs if you end your run too suddenly. This can cause dizziness and fainting. A gradual slowdown reduces the strain on your cardiovascular system and allows the leg muscles to keep pumping blood back up to your heart. You'll also help your muscles rid themselves of the lactic acid (the waste produced by muscles as they burn fuel) they've built up over the course of your run. Letting the lactic acid remain in your muscles will contribute to muscle soreness.

Allow 8 minutes at the end of your run for your cool-down. Start by alternating 30 to 60 seconds of slow jogging with the same amount of walking for a total of 5 minutes, and then walk the final 3 minutes. Keep in mind that the harder you run, the more time you should devote to your cool-down.

## ...AND STRETCH

Stretching helps keep your muscles and joints supple, and the flexibility it provides protects you from injury. Even when your muscles are tight, the care you take performing a stretch properly puts you in a calm, meditative state of mind—another reward for your time and effort. The key is to stretch properly—we show you how on pages 40 through 46.

When should you stretch? After you run, sometimes during, but *never* before. Many athletes make the mistake of stretching before they have warmed up, which can strain cold muscles to the tearing point at worst, or leave you feeling wobbly at best. If you feel yourself tightening up during a run, or if you enjoy stretching for a few minutes after your warm-up, take a few moments to do so, but then get back into your workout as soon as possible so that you don't cool down prematurely. In brief, think of stretching as your post-workout reward—the soothing release from a good hard effort.

## STRETCHING GUIDELINES

Before you begin, keep in mind these simple rules for keeping your stretching session safe and effective:

**Make it routine** Make stretching an integral part of your workout, not a supplement you sometimes make time for, sometimes not.

**Take it slow** Ease into any stretch very slowly. The body tenses muscles after the first two to three seconds of stretching; slowly easing into a pose allows you to work with this reflex, not against it.

**Don't force it** Never stretch to the point of pain. Mild discomfort should be your stopping point. Depending on your level of flexibility, you may experience relaxation from stretching, as opposed to discomfort.

**Hold it** Once you're in a stretch, hold it for 10 to 20 seconds, breathing deeply to help you relax into it, then release gradually.

**Don't bounce** Bouncing during a stretch can hyperextend muscles and joints, leading to injury.

Remember that increasing your flexibility requires commitment over time; results will come from your frequent stretch breaks, not from occasional post-run stretching.

# Full Body Stretch Circuit

What follows is a stretching circuit—a group of stretches that you can perform at the end of your run and cooldown. Make sure to follow the stretching guidelines on the previous pages. Hold each stretch for 10 to 20 seconds and then move onto the next one. Remember: Never force a stretch to the point of pain. If you're not able to reach or stretch as far as our models, do what you're able to and work up to the full stretch.

## HAMSTRING STRETCH

With your legs straight, bend forward from the hips and reach for your toes with your outstretched arms. Hold, then draw yourself back up slowly, vertebra by vertebra, using your abdominal muscles to ease any strain you may feel in your lower back. You don't need to actually reach your toes for this stretch to be effective.

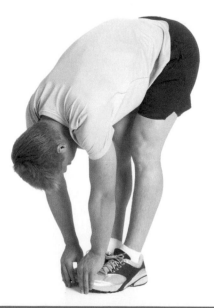

## CALF STRETCH

Stand roughly 2 feet from a wall with your feet about 6 inches apart. Lean in and place your palms on the wall. Lean forward from your hips, keeping your heels flat on the ground. You should feel the stretch in your calf muscles.

## QUAD STRETCH

Grab your left foot with your left hand. While keeping the thigh muscles of your right leg tight, pull your left knee back and up toward your buttocks. For balance, rest your right hand on a wall, tree, or fence. Do not tilt forward.

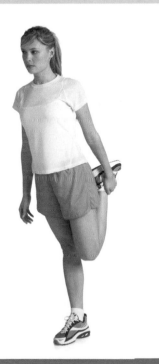

## GROIN STRETCH

While seated on the floor with your back straight, pull your legs into a diamond shape in front of you, with the soles of your feet touching (your knees will be splayed out to the side like butterfly wings). Lean forward from the hip, grasp your ankles, and use your elbows to press your knees down until you feel a stretch in your groin muscles. Hold, and release.

## MODIFIED HURDLER STRETCH

While seated, extend your right leg in front of you. Bend your left leg and place the sole of your left foot against the inside of your right thigh. Slowly reach forward with your arms toward your right knee or toes, taking care to bend from the hips. This pose stretches nearly everything in your right leg, up your back and down your right arm. Hold, release by sitting upright, switch legs and repeat on the other side of your body

## LOWER BACK STRETCH

Lie flat on your back with your arms extended to the sides. Bend your legs and bring your knees up and over your hips. Gently drop your legs over to the right side, allowing your lower trunk to twist to the right while your shoulders remain firmly planted on the floor. Hold, then ease out of this stretch by extending your legs back out (rather than pulling them back up over your hips), and repeat on the left side.

## ILIOTIBIAL BAND STRETCH

Remain lying on your back, legs extended in front of you, with your arms stretched out to either side. Keep your shoulders and arms flat on the floor. Lift your right leg slightly and cross it over your body to the left by rolling at the hip, keeping your legs fully extended. You may or may not be able to touch the floor with the toes of your right foot, but at any rate they should be tending downwards, with your right heel pointed correspondingly up. Hold, return your right leg to a resting position alongside your left, and repeat the stretch with your left leg.

## BUTT AND AB TWIST

Sit upright with your feet flat on the ground. Cross your left leg over your right, placing your left foot on the right side of your right knee. Twist your torso to the left while keeping your spine straight. Brace your twist with your right arm, which should extend down from your shoulder along the line of your left shin, so that your right elbow touches the outside of your left knee. Look over your left shoulder to avoid straining your neck, and breathe normally. Hold, release by twisting your torso back to center, then switch to the other leg.

## STRADDLE STRETCH

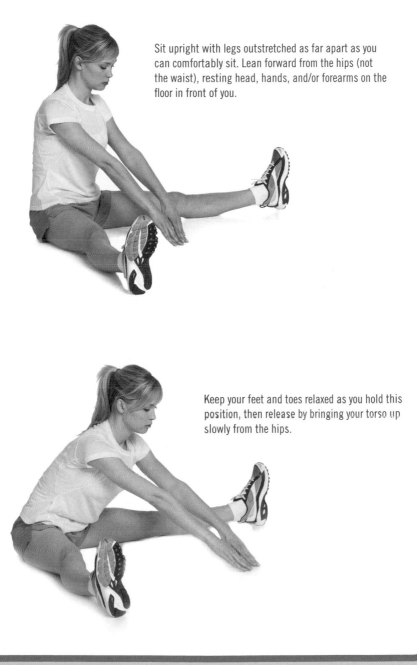

Sit upright with legs outstretched as far apart as you can comfortably sit. Lean forward from the hips (not the waist), resting head, hands, and/or forearms on the floor in front of you.

Keep your feet and toes relaxed as you hold this position, then release by bringing your torso up slowly from the hips.

## A FINAL NOTE ON STRETCHING

Need more convincing that stretching before running is not a good idea? A recent study found that stretching before an activity actually slows performance. When your muscles are relatively tight, you get the springy stride you need for fast running. On the other hand, stretching after your activity provides myriad benefits. Flexible muscles and joints are less likely to be injured by a misstep and stretching helps regulate imbalances between opposing muscles. In other words, if you maintain flexibility, your body is better able to mitigate the effects of, for instance, hamstrings that are better developed than the quadriceps.

Keep in mind stretching is no substitute for a proper warm-up. Transitioning from walking to your running pace increases your heart rate and body temperature; stretching before a run actually delays this physiological transition. That also means you should warm up before stretching on any non-running days. Bouncing while you stretch, known as ballistic stretching, is not only unhelpful, but it could be harmful to your muscles. Stretch and hold gently for up to 30 seconds for the best results.

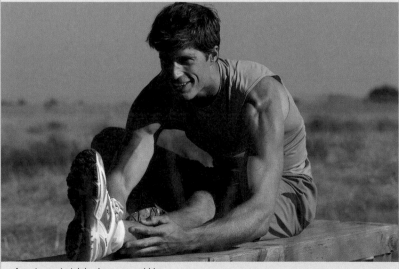

A post-run stretch is always a good idea.

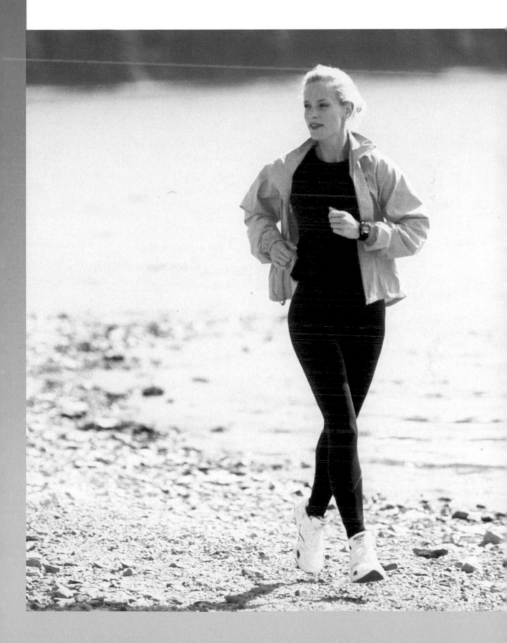

# PART III:
# THE RUNNING PLANS

# On Your Mark

This might be your first try at running, a return visit, or an attempt to improve your current running performance. The less running you've done recently, the more you can expect to improve your distances and speeds in the next 10 weeks. That's the good news. The bad news is the less you've run lately, the more likely you are to run a lot more than you should when you first start a new running program, resulting in possible injury. That's why it's important to set two related goals as you start your running program: Maximize improvements and minimize injuries. You win by improving, and you lose by getting hurt. Remember this principle as you move forward.

What else do you need to keep in mind? While by no means exhaustive, this laundry list of topics will give you an overview of some of the most important principles:

**Buy the right shoes** We've discussed shoes at length in Part II, so we won't belabor the point, except to say that a good pair of shoes should carry you 400 to 500 miles (640 km to 800 km) before you need to replace them.

**Lose the excuses** The two most basic elements of a running routine are time and space. And the two main reasons given by people who don't run? "I don't have time for it" and "I don't have anywhere to do it." Let's dissect those excuses. You can run well and get in great shape with a modest time investment of 1 half-hour every other day. Think of it as time you won't waste watching television.

As for finding places to run, anywhere that's safe for walking is safe for running. Off-road routes (parks, bike paths, school tracks) are better than high-traffic streets, and soft surfaces like dirt or grass are better than pavement, but any choice is better than staying at home. Start by mapping out four or five courses in your immediate neighborhood—it saves time, solves the "place" issue, and increases the likelihood that you'll follow through on your planned runs. And don't be tempted to do your mapping by car, either; walking these routes before you run is the best preparation, as it both acquaints you intimately

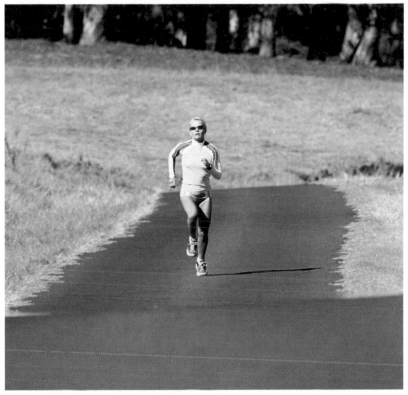

Running can be just the break you need to clear your mind.

with the geography of your route and helps prepare you physically for the runs to follow (although you may have to measure distance by car).

**Run safely at all times** If you're running on a road, run facing oncoming traffic, so that you're always able to see what's coming; and obey traffic signs, signals, and every other rule of the road, that way drivers can trust that you're predictable in your actions. Never forget that every moving car deserves your wariness and attention. And depending upon where you workout, it may be a good idea to run with friends.

**Listen to your body** Most running injuries are self-inflicted, caused by running too much too soon or other improper training methods. The best prevention you can practice is to pay attention to the signals from your body, and modify your routine as needed. Let pain guide you away from the bad and toward the good.

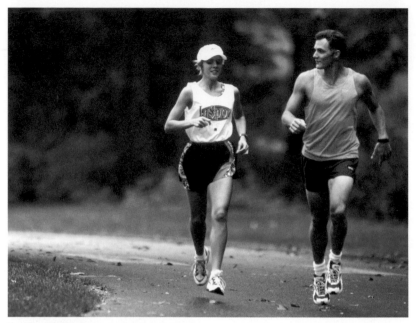

If you can't talk during a run, slow down your pace.

## TAKE THE TALK TEST

For beginning runners eager to get started but without the benefit of experience in pacing themselves, the talk test is a great tool. In short, if you can't hold a conversation with someone while running, you're running too fast. The talk test is an immediate barometer of the pressure you're putting on yourself in a run. Can't talk? Just slow it down a bit and enjoy your run and your company.

The best advice for new runners about breathing is to not worry about it too much; just breathe any way that gets air into your lungs. Don't force yourself to breathe through your nose entirely or in a complicated "in-through-the-nose, out-through-the-mouth" routine. Stay relaxed by breathing deeply and fully. For many people, the result will be something even and regular: One inhalation over the course of two to three steps, then an exhalation over the next two to three steps.

For harder runs and uphill stretches (which you should avoid for the first several months of your training program), you may wish to intentionally alter your breathing pattern to accommodate the extra effort you're making. Try this technique: inhale for two steps, and exhale for one step. Inhalation should be smooth and easy, and the exhalation should be shorter and more forceful. This method can help to prevent cramps and keep you from gasping for air.

## TRY OUT THE TREADMILL

Contrary to what you might think, treadmills are neither a poor excuse for the great outdoors nor ideal substitutes for the rigors of more varied running surfaces. For some people, they just work, and you have nothing to lose by starting your running program on one if it's your only option. In fact, treadmills have the following advantages:

The smooth, rotating belt and forgiving running surface provided by a treadmill cushions your feet, which results in less stress being placed on your joints. That leads to more effortless (and enjoyable) running, a boon for runners who are overweight or who are otherwise worried about such issues.

Treadmills are almost always found indoors, so you can run at any time of day, regardless of the conditions outside.

Most models are programmable, so you can set up your entire workout (different speeds and/or grades of the running surface) ahead of time.

Are you a runner who enjoys getting into a mental zone and staying there? The treadmill might be just the training tool you're looking for. But if you like distractions as you run, a treadmill might also be your best bet. It's much safer to strap on your portable MP3 player, and turn up the volume while running indoors. If you're at home, you can listen to your stereo or even watch television. If you want to strip your running experience down to the essentials, there's no better way to do it than climbing on and punching "start."

## ⟫ I WISH I HAD KNOWN . . .

"You need to enjoy the running experience if you want to continue and succeed at it. But this can take time. You need to be patient. Running doesn't always jump out at you as the greatest thing since sliced bread. Eventually though, you realize it is."

—Jack, age 68
Years running: 45

# Time to Train

Now you're ready to start your training. Here you'll find two programs—The 30/30 Plan and The 10-Week Run/ Walk Plan. Use the plans consecutively and in approximately 3½ months, you'll be running 20 minutes at least three times a week. But first, we look at why walking and running are not mutually exclusive in a runner's workout.

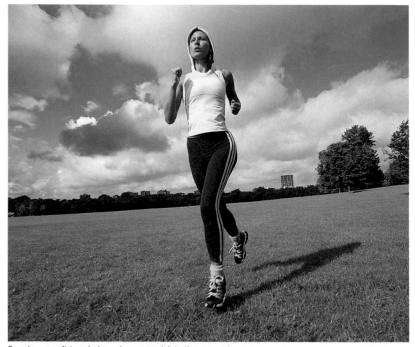

Running on soft terrain is easier on your joints than concrete.

You may feel that you won't be a real runner until you can run a set time or distance without walking. But it's time to adjust your expectations. Not only will combining running and walking reduce your chances of injury and enable you to increase the length of your workouts (and therefore improve your performance), it will make you a more successful runner.

In the not so distant past, advice for beginning runners could have been distilled to five words:

Start running, and don't stop. Slowing down was permissible, but stopping or walking was tantamount to failure. Beginning runners suffered needless pain, injuries, and even emotional distress as a result. Worse, many gave up and returned to their sedentary ways.

The missing component in their training was walking. Not simply because walking provides an essential breather no matter your fitness level, but because walking and running complement each other so perfectly. Working out at both intensities will build your overall level of fitness better than doing just one or the other.

That's quite a claim to make, but the daily experience of thousands of runners bears it out. Marathoners and ultramarathoners routinely include walk breaks in their training and races. Intermediate and advanced runners alternate intense running with walking or jogging "recovery" periods—what's known as interval training—to increase speed and endurance. The common denominator in these examples is, of course, continuous movement, rather than constant velocity. "Run/walk" has become the shorthand expression for this kinder, gentler, and smarter way to train, and it is the key to becoming the runner you want to be.

## TWO SIDES, SAME COIN

It's worth a moment to draw out the similarities and differences between running and walking. If you've ever walked as fast as you could without breaking into a run, you've approached the crossover

## IS IT GOING TOO WELL?

You have your plan, you've laced your shoes, and you hit the road. Despite your expectations, you're able to run farther than you imagined, and you're having a hard time stopping yourself. While it may seem odd to talk about overtraining this early in your running career, it's a risk for runners at every level. Remember, the key to running success is gradual adaptation. Ramping up your time spent running slowly is the key, or you may waste time with an injury caused by over-zealous training. This is particularly a problem for new runners. Stick to your plan—it's the safest way to get where you want to go.

point: the "jump" that runners make from foot to foot. No matter how fast they go, even professional speed walkers always keep one foot on the ground at all times, whereas runners get a little air with every stride.

What does that little jump entail? A bigger flex to the knee, greater contraction of the quadriceps muscles, and the all-important *toe off* action, where the toe of your foot pushes your leg forward toward the next stride. After you toe off, you land rather forcefully on your other foot. Often described as the "impact shock" of running, your feet alternate taking on the pressure of two to three times your body weight. Even if you're a daily walker, your joints, tendons, and ligaments need time to adapt to the increased impact shock of running—hence, the usefulness of the run/walk system.

At this point, you may be asking why anyone runs at all, given the stress on your body impact shock can cause. But your body adapts quickly to and benefits from the rigors of running. From a calorie-burning perspective, you move a lot faster while running, and this leads to a higher caloric burn. Burning more calories more quickly equals a more time-efficient workout, which is a real benefit in our hectic, multitasked, over-scheduled world.

You can incorporate training with other runners at many different levels. Want to go for a run with the whole family, but you know not everyone can do a full half-hour of continuous running? Enter run/walk. Keep it easy, conversational, and involve everyone in setting the pace.

You truly have nothing to lose and everything to gain by giving run/walk a try. The three workouts

## >> I WISH I HAD KNOWN . . .

"When I started running in my mid-20s, I thought running on a treadmill was cheating, so I'd push myself to head out on the worst days. Now I realize that I can sometimes get a better quality workout on the treadmill."

—David, age 41
*Years running: 16*

in this book—the 30/30 Plan for base running fitness, and the 10-Week Run/Walk Plan—utilize this basic formula for great results, and the speed work introduction in *"Reaching the Next Level: Speed Work"* takes run/walk to the next level. Get your running off to the right start with run/walk.

## THE 30/30 PLAN

This running plan is simplicity itself. It contains all the elements you need in an all-in-one workout for beginners—a warm-up, a cool-down, and a middle phase during which you do your most vigorous activity. In contrast to some other running plans, it also sports a recommended time frame for its use: the first 30 days of your new life as a runner. After a month with the 30/30 plan, you will have a great fitness base from which to strive for the next level.

To start, map out a 30-minute route for yourself. You may want to map out a few in your vicinity, so that you can enjoy a diversity of different locales.

When you start your workout, walk for the first 10 minutes. Even if you're tempted to break into a run, stick with walking. The same goes for the

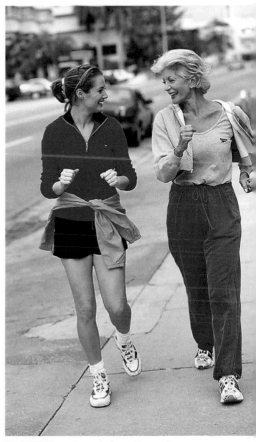

The 30/30 Plan gets your body used to—and comfortable with—running.

last 5 minutes of your workout: Just walk. The 15 minutes in the middle are yours to divide between walking and jogging or—only if you're able to comfortably—jogging and running. No matter how you move, keep it to a pace during which you can talk comfortably. Most important is that whatever you choose should feel enjoyable.

For your first few workouts, try jogging for 30 seconds, then walking until you feel ready to jog for another 30 seconds, and so on for the entire 15-minute period.

Soon you'll feel your stamina increase. When that happens, gradually shift to a ratio of 30 seconds of jogging, followed by 30 seconds of walking, then back to jogging, and so on. You may find yourself wanting to depart from a 30/30 ratio in favor of 60-second intervals or longer; resist the temptation. Remember that the 30/30 Plan is designed to let your body gradually get used to running; though your mind may feel ready to run for longer stretches, your muscles and joints need your continued patience.

Thirty consecutive days of 30/30 workouts will get you to the point where you're covering 1 to 2 miles daily, and you'll be ready to take on the next challenge. If you feel that every other day would suit you better, you'll complete the 30/30 Plan in two months. Either way, remember that the point of this plan is to allow your body to adapt to running; take your time and listen to your body so you won't be tempted to overtrain; that will only lead to injury.

## THE 10-WEEK RUN/WALK PLAN

Congratulations—you've completed the 30/30 Plan. If you're not already surprised by the progress you've made, you soon will be. The *Runner's World* 10-week Run/Walk program is specifically designed to take you to the next level in your running life.

The American College of Sports Medicine (ACSM) has determined that with only 20 minutes of continuous running, three to four times a week, you will accrue the most important benefits of an exercise program: increased cardiovascular health, weight loss, increased muscle strength, and stress reduction, among others. At *Runner's World*, we don't stress continuous running so much as continuous movement, so keep in mind that pace is not important. Combined with a warm-up and cool-down (see pages 36–39 for recommendations), this program will deliver the health benefits you seek while building your endurance as a runner.

During each week, do the run/walk combination three or four times. Your lifestyle will dictate which days of the week work best for you, but here are two sample schedules:

- Run on Monday, Wednesday, and Friday, and fit in a fourth run on either Saturday or Sunday (whichever day works best for you—just maintain consistency to help build a strong habit).
- Run on Tuesday, Thursday, Saturday and Sunday.

## THE 10-PERCENT SOLUTION

It's one of the most important rules of running—whether you're a beginner or an elite athlete: Increase your weekly time or distance spent running by *no more than 10 percent over the previous week's training*. That means if you ran 10 miles (16.9 km) last week—and assuming you *want* to increase your mileage—you should run no more than 11 miles (18.59 km) this week. If you ran 120 minutes (4 days x 30 minutes) last week, you should run for no more than 132 minutes (4 days x 33 minutes) this week.

As a beginner, you may chafe at this requirement. "But my body is ready to go further," you insist. Trust us: Bide your time. Your body requires time to gradually become accustomed to the rigors or running. If you push yourself

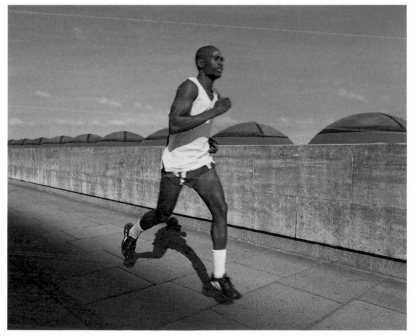

Even marathoners don't increase their mileage more than 10 percent a week—and neither should you.

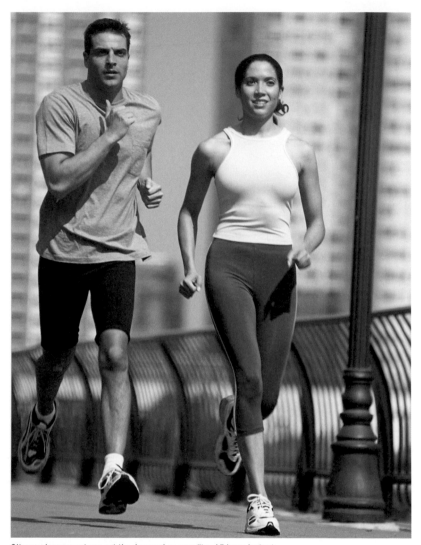

City running can get you out the door and on your "track" in an instant.

too hard in the beginning you are more likely to sustain an injury that can hinder the rest of your running experience. The mental discipline you're building now will serve you well later in your running career.

## THE PLAN

If, during Week Ten, you find that you can't run continuously for 20 minutes, that's fine. You'll see from the chart that we're assuming your stamina for longer

## 10-WEEK RUN/WALK PLAN

| Week | Run | Walk | Repeat | Total Time |
|------|------|------|--------|------------|
| 1 | 1 min | 2 min | 7x | 21 min |
| 2 | 1 min | 1 min | 10x | 20 min |
| 3 | 2 min | 1 min | 7x | 21 min |
| 4 | 3 min | 1 min | 5x | 20 min |
| 5 | 4 min | 1 min | 4x | 20 min |
| 6 | 6 min | 1 min | 3x | 21 min |
| 7 | 9 min | 1 min | 2x | 20 min |
| 8 | 12 min | 1 min | Then run 7 min | 20 min |
| 9 | 15 min | 1 min | Then run 4 min | 20 min |
| 10 | 20 min | Leap for joy | — | 20 min |

runs is growing ever greater from week to week, but your individual stamina curve may be different. Instead of pushing yourself unduly toward that 20-minute goal, go back and run the Week seven workout. The following week, run a modification of the Week eight workout: 12 minutes running, 1 to 2 minutes walking, and then repeat. You're still building endurance, thanks to the interval-like training those walking breaks give you.

When you're ready, try for 20 minutes of continuous running again, and if it still eludes you, modify the Week nine workout just as you did for Week eight: Run 15 minutes, walk for 1 to 2 minutes, then repeat. Keep attempting to reach your 20-minute goal once a week. Stick with a modified Week nine schedule, increasing your minutes of continuous running gradually by 1 or 2 additional minutes. In short order, you will have achieved the 20-minute goal, and you'll have gained valuable experience at modifying a plan to suit your individual abilities.

A final note: Resist the temptation to run on your "days off"—these are your rest days, and good rest is as important to your running performance as dedication, nutritious food, and the right shoes. If you must get in some sort of physical activity, try an easy walk with a friend. The conversation will take the pressure off, but you will burn off that excess energy all the same.

# Easing into Speed Work

Once you're able to run for 20 to 30 minutes at least three times a week, it's a good idea to hold there for a couple of months before trying to increase your pace. This will give your body an opportunity to get stronger and to adapt to your new active lifestyle.

After that, though, you may find that you've hit a plateau–having reached a certain level of fitness, only to find yourself stuck there. Runners at all levels experience plateaus, but speed work can help you get over them, while increasing your strength and endurance.

Here are four speed workouts. Do them one at a time and in the order in which they're presented, for a 4-week speed work program. Note: Do not try to increase your speed and distance at the same time. Maintain your weekly distance for the 4 weeks of this program. Beginners should limit speed workouts to once a week.

**Strides** (or pickups) are accelerations of your pace for short distances toward the end of your regular run. The goal of striding is to teach you to run in a "fast-but-relaxed" way with good form. As you complete your run, find a smooth stretch of road or grass 100 to 150 meters (110 to 165 yds) long. For the first 30 to 50 meters (32 to 54 yds), gradually accelerate to nearly top speed, and then hold that pace for 50 to 75 meters (54 to 82 yards) before gradually decelerating. Recover for 1 minute with an easy jog. This is one stride. Run six to ten strides, stopping as soon as you feel yourself straining.

**Out-and-backs** are a way of organizing your run so that halfway through your course, you turn around and return to your starting point at a slightly faster pace. Map out a relatively flat course, and take note of your usual time at the turnaround point. On the return leg, strive for a pace that is 20 to 40 seconds per kilometer (30 to 60 seconds per mi) faster than your pace on the first portion of the run. You should be working slightly harder on the return trip, but not so hard that you end up exhausted and unable to jog.

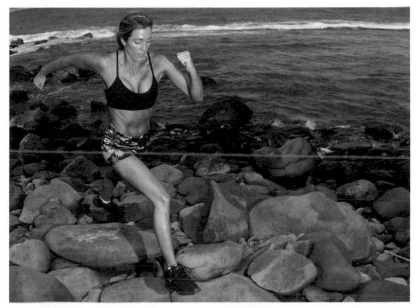

Speed work can help make reaching the next level a less rocky road.

**Continuous 400s** are runs during which you change your pace every 100 meters (110 yds) from a walk to a jog to a striding pace to what's called *race pace*: A fast, high-effort pace characterized by quick leg turnover. Best performed on a stretch of grass, road, or trail that is about 400 meters long (approximately a quarter-mile), continuous 400s should be run without stopping, and without sprinting during the striding or race pace portions. Repeat this cycle four times, gradually working your way up to six or more in each session.

**Cruise intervals** are short, fast runs followed by jogging recoveries. Cruise intervals are run at a "fast-but-controlled" speed: a pace you can hold for 4 to 6 minutes that leaves you tired but not exhausted. The first time you try this speed exercise, warm up, then run a 4- to 6-minute interval followed by a 2-minute jog. Repeat this cycle up to three times. As your strength increases, increase the length of your cruise interval up to 10 minutes, and/or shorten the duration of your jog afterward. Either way, limit your cruise interval workout to 40 minutes total.

Dedicate just 5 percent of your training to speed work—6 minutes a week if your total running time is 2 hours—you'll start to see the benefits after just a few sessions.

# All-in-One Workout

For whatever the reason—it's the holidays and your time is very limited, you haven't organized your training week well and you need to get the essentials in, or you just want to take all the guesswork out of your workout—you'll appreciate the following run. It's basic, and if you're able to run continuously for 20 minutes (the goal of the *Runner's World* 10-week Run/Walk Plan), you can do this one without any additional special training. You can even do this workout on a treadmill.

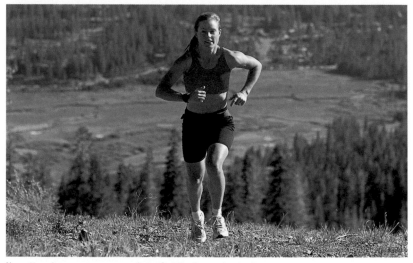

No matter where you are, you can always find the time and space to run.

To complete the workout, move from Part I to Part II to Part III without stopping. In total, the workout should take you approximately 40 minutes.

## PART I: GEAR-SHIFTERS

- 1st gear: Warm up for 10 minutes with an easy walk/jog.
- 2nd gear: Run for 30 seconds at a pace that is slightly faster than your warm-up pace.
- 3rd gear: Run for 30 seconds more at a slightly accelerated pace.
- 4th gear: Run for 60 seconds at your cruise interval pace, fast-but-controlled (see page 61). Remember, this is not a sprint pace, but a race pace.

- 3rd gear: Shift down to 3rd gear for 30 seconds.
- 2nd gear: Reduce your speed again, to 2nd gear, for 30 seconds.

You've just run through all the gears in 3 minutes. Repeat the cycle immediately.

## PART II: HILL RUNS

- Run up a moderate hill for 40 to 50 meters at a medium-hard effort, then recover by jogging or walking slowly back down the hill. Repeat for a total of 8 minutes.

## PART III: GEAR-SHIFTERS

- Do two more Gear-Shifter Drills.
- Cool down for 10 minutes as you would normally.

This is an intense and powerful workout, and the same two maxims apply here as they do in all of the other workouts we recommend: (1) Don't run through pain—slow down or stop before you injure yourself; and (2) walking is just fine if it helps you keep going through the workout.

Keep in mind that all the terms we use here are relative. If you have been running for only 4 months, you may not be able to run as fast as a friend who has been running for years. Work hard, but stay within your capabilities.

## CUTTING BACK

As you progress further in your career as a runner, it's a good idea to cut back on your training for one week every couple of months to recharge your body. This time off will not result in a decrease in fitness, but rather an improvement. How much should you cut back? About 50 percent. Let's say you normally run 20 miles each week. During your cut-down week, reduce that amunt to 10 miles. Use your training log (see page 81) to help you build a schedule that includes a cut-down week. If you find yourself getting antsy during your low-mileage weeks, incorporate some easy cross-training into your schedule. Remember, the goal of this week is to reduce your training, not simply exchange one kind of workout for another. You'll return the next week with more energy, a stronger body, and increased commitment to your running practice.

# Avoiding Injury

All runners experience aches and pains now and then, but usually these fall under the heading of "temporary discomforts": they go away in a few days, provided you take some appropriate steps (more on that below). Serious injuries, however, require much more care, and like the broken axle on your car that followed a persistent noise that you ignored, they can sometimes develop from small discomforts that you neglect.

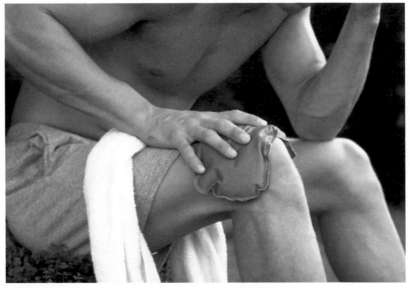

Paying attention to minor discomfort now can save you from serious injury later.

For optimum running health, you should follow some basic guidelines to keep from getting hurt and to treat yourself appropriately before injuries grow too serious.

## THE BASIC TENETS

Follow these rules of running and you'll greatly decrease your chances of being sidelined by injury.

**Increase duration gradually** Your body needs time to adapt to running if you want to enjoy a long running career. This means not increasing your time spent running by more than 10 percent a week (See *The 10-Percent Solution*, page 57).

**Increase intensity gradually** Just as you gradually increase the amount of time or distance that you run, it's vital to do the same with your intensity, or speed. Faster running places greater strain on the body, which means your muscles work harder and suffer more (temporary) damage, your joints absorb greater impact, and your body expends more energy overall. The result: Your body needs more time to adjust to this increased load. Increasing the intensity of your workouts too soon can do more harm than good.

**Increase distance before speed** For beginners who have just enjoyed week after week of improvement, it's easy to want to increase distance and pace at the same time. That's a recipe for injury. A solid base of running at easy, slow speeds is essential before you build speed work into your workouts. What's a solid base? Complete both the 30/30 Plan and the *Runner's World* 10-Week Run/Walk Plan, then work your way up to running 4 to 5 days a week consistently for several months—then it's safe to begin speed training.

**Rest after hard runs** We've highlighted the importance of rest in a general sense, but you should always take a day off after a difficult run. Your muscles and joints need time to repair themselves, and they won't get it if you hit the streets again right away.

**Heed early warning signs** All-over aches and minor discomfort come with the territory when you're starting out, and you'll experience them again when you increase the intensity

## ≫ I WISH I HAD KNOWN . . .

"Taking care of myself and staying uninjured is more important than any training run or race. If I'd figured that out last winter when I rolled my ankle badly, I would've taken the time to get better, even though it would've meant skipping the Boston Marathon. Instead, I tried to train through it and made the injury worse. So I missed Boston—and months of training along with it. I've made a solemn vow to never do that again. You must be patient and smart about injury recovery."

*—Parker, age 26*
*Years running: 14*

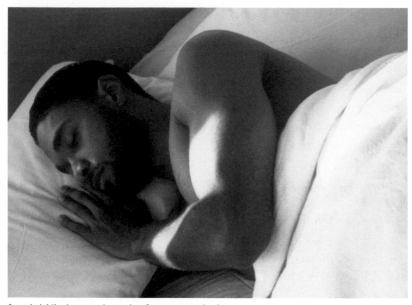

A good night's sleep can do wonders for your energy level.

of your training. Generally, these are nothing to worry about. But sharp localized pains, especially in your joints, are red flags. If they occur suddenly and/or get worse during a run, slow down or stop. Return home, taking the shortest route possible. Try to run the next day, but if you encounter swelling and/or the pain returns, skip your run and check out our recommendations on page 84–87.

**Wear the right shoes** If you haven't already read *Gearing Up,* (pages 25 to 27) about choosing the right running shoes, do it now. Your awareness of how your body feels during and after your workouts is your first line of injury defense, but your shoes are a close second. If you're wearing the wrong kind or they're worn out, it's time for a new pair.

**Cross-train** It's worth stressing how effective other physical activities, especially low-weight strength training, cycling, and swimming are, for strengthening your body.

**Stretch and strengthen** Regular running can tighten your muscles, leading to reduced range of motion and poor form. This in turn, can place added stress on your body, and lead to injuries. You can break the vicious cycle by always including a stretching routine in your training to lengthen and strengthen your muscles. See pages 40 to 45 for a sample stretching program.

**Run a variety of routes and surfaces** Wise runners mix it up on both counts, and their ankles benefit from it. Concrete and tarmac are especially tough on your feet, and inclined roads can place unequal stresses on legs. The solution: Get off the road and onto grass, trails, cinder paths or even dirt whenever you can. Sandy beaches and grassy parks are great for building flexibility in your feet and ankles, and the soft surfaces absorb impact so your body doesn't have to.

**Feed your body** Dehydration and lack of the right types of food will negatively impact your running in many ways, making it both more difficult to complete your workout and to return to full strength afterwards. Drink up and fuel up for success. (See *Eat and Drink Right* on pages 30 to 35 for more information about what and how to eat and drink to improve your running performance.)

## LISTEN TO YOUR BODY

At the first sign of persistent pain, stop training for 3 days, and ice the sore area twice a day for 10 to 15 minutes at a time.

During this period, resist the urge to stretch your injury; a partially-torn muscle or aggravated joint can actually be injured further by trying to stretch it out.

Over-the-counter anti-inflammatories such as ibuprofen can also be effective at reducing swelling and any pain you may experience. After 3 days, start training again slowly—a walk is a great way to start—and assess yourself sensibly. If the pain returns, contact a physical therapist or sports medicine practitioner for some professional advice.

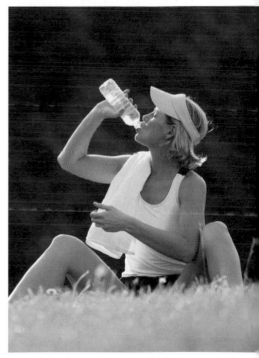

Staying hydrated is one way to ward off injury.

## SHINSPLINTS

Few running injuries seem to be as universally bemoaned as shinsplints. A better name for the condition might be "tendonitis of the shin," since the condition occurs when tendons along the shin get strained. The most common, and almost always preventable, causes of shinsplints include:

- Increasing distance too quickly. In other words, heed the 10 percent rule (See page 57).
- Worn-out shoes. A visit to the running shoe store can solve this problem.
- Overpronation (see pages 24 to 27). If you overpronate, ask a running shoe store staff member about shoes that will correct the condition.
- A sudden switch from running mostly on grass or trails to running on concrete or tarmac or vice versa. Increase your time on the harder surfaces gradually—literally just a few minutes during each run—to avoid this pitfall.
- Overly tight or weak calf muscles. Stretching your shin and calf muscles dutifully after each run, preferably as part of a regular post-run stretching routine, will lengthen and strengthen your lower legs over time. Check out the section on pages 40 to 45 for stretches that target this area.

The inflammation, tenderness, and pain of shinsplints will plague you most before and after your run, when your muscles are cold, so look for this tell-tale sign. Treatment is simple: Take a few days off from running, ice and massage the area, and stretch very gently. If you like, cross train in another sport until you're ready to run again. If your shinsplints haven't disappeared within two weeks, see a doctor.

# PART IV:
# GETTING OUT

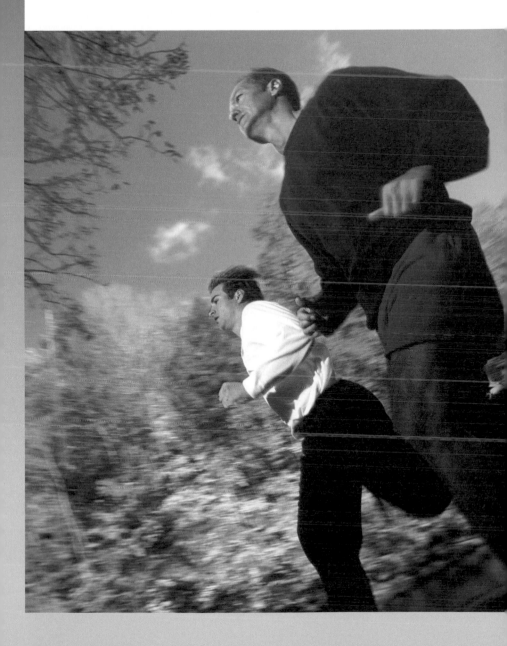

# Social Running

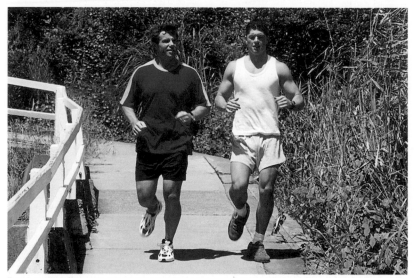

Running with a friend can provide you with motivation and support to stick to any running plan.

Running with others is one of the best steps you can take to strengthen your commitment to running. Whether you join a running club or the weekly group run starting from your local shoe store; whether you set up a standing running date with a friend, or just try a new way to bond with your dog, social running connects you with others who share your interest in the sport.

Even if you are a confirmed solo runner, you owe it to yourself to investigate running with others. The benefits of running in groups are countless and well worth exploring.

**Stress reduction** As soon as you start running with a friend, the conversations begin and the stress disappears like morning fog in bright sunlight. You'll cover *more* ground *more* easily, and enjoy it *more*.

**Training variety** Some running partners are naturally faster than you, others slower. Challenge yourself with your faster friends on days when you want a harder workout, and recover with your slower friends.

**A stronger commitment**
When you know someone is waiting for you—at the park, on the corner, at the gym—you're not as likely to skip that day's run at the last minute. Running with others means it's not just about you anymore. The social element is a strong motivator, and your commitment to others can sometimes be more of a driving force than your commitment to yourself.

**Co-opetition** Okay, we'll admit it, we made up that word. But most people can't help feeling a bit competitive with their running buddy, even though you rely on that person's presence and encouragement to keep you going. Undoubtedly, your buddy feels the same mix of feelings toward you. Nurture that push-and-pull so that you both become stronger runners. Competition and cooperation equal co-opetition.

**Safety** It may not be a jungle out there where you live and run, but let's face it—accidents can happen. Be it a running partner or a posse at your side,

## RUNNING WITH YOUR PARTNER OR SPOUSE

It might seem like the ultimate combination—a good run with that special someone at the center of your life—and it can be, provided you take extra care to make things pleasant and fair. Whereas you might not care if your running buddy from down the street starts to achieve Olympian greatness, you might feel more than a twinge of abandonment if your spouse does. So keep your runs together lighthearted and fun if you're just starting to workout.

Try alternating who's in charge of the content and pacing of your workouts, and keep the lines of communication open. For some couples, running together provides an outlet for the competitive or aggressive feelings that might be difficult to work through in other ways; for other couples, running together strengthens their emotional bonds and intensifies their physical attraction for one another. In any event, recognize that when you run with the love of your life, you're working out on more than one level, which may take some getting used to. With the right steps and the right attitude, you should both feel closer as a result.

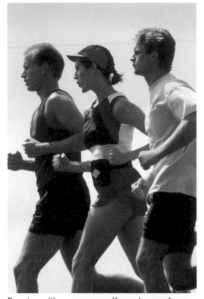

Running with a group can offer a change of pace.

you're better protected from danger, and you can venture farther afield and at odder hours than you'd feel comfortable doing alone. And should you fall and twist your ankle, you have someone with you who can help you hobble home or even call for help if necessary.

**Confidence** When you run with others, you validate your status as a runner in your own mind. Beginners, and those returning to the sport, can sometimes feel like interlopers. If you've ever felt unsure about describing yourself as a runner, this is the easiest route to assurance. Find a community of

runners or build it one buddy at a time, and you'll soon feel like the runner you already are.

## FIND A RUNNING BUDDY

If you're one of the lucky ones with a long list of running buddies, count your blessings. Some runners, especially beginners, keenly feel the isolation of running solo, despite the pleasures of getting out there and doing it all by themselves. Here are some tips for finding the fleet friends who will change your running experiences for the better.

**Ask friends and acquaintances** The runner in your social circle should be the first person you chat with about heading out for a run together. Social runs are a great way to get to know someone better, especially if your respective training levels mesh well. If it doesn't work out, don't be discouraged. Ask around in your social circle to find other runners whose training stage, goals, and pace might be more in sync with yours.

**Include your family** You may already be sharing a roof with the best running buddies you could hope to find. Make a running date with your partner, but pay close attention to your respective paces and levels of fitness, so that you're not introducing unnecessary tension. Adolescent and teenage children may be more or less willing to explore running with you, depending on your relationship with them; with the proper approach, your workouts could provide a new avenue for bonding. The trick with family running partners is to let steadfast training goals take a backseat to good dynamics. Go for fun and inclusiveness above all.

**Take a four-footed friend** You've seen them on the trail and in the park, and now you're wondering what it is about running with a dog that is so appealing. Dogs, like people, need daily exercise to feel their best, and some breeds just love to run. It takes training to bring a dog "up to speed"—you'll need to start with short runs, building distance gradually as your pet's stamina builds. Age and temperament can play a role in your ultimate success, and no dog owner would deny the hard work that raising a dog can sometimes be. Talk to runners who regularly train with their canine friends to learn from their experiences.

## GROUP RUNS

If you've never run with a group before, you're in for a real treat. At its best, group running delivers a feeling of camaraderie, support, and even a sense of team spirit, that is rare for those of us who aren't members of rock bands or rugby squads.

When you work out with other runners, you're participating in an experience that goes back to the beginnings of humanity,

>> **I WISH I HAD KNOWN...**

"I'd taken years off from running when I had children, so when I started up again, I felt so slow that I was too embarrassed to run with anyone else. That was a mistake. Finally when I started training for the Philadelphia (USA) Half-Marathon, I joined a group for long runs on weekends. Being in a group motivated me tremendously, and made 10 miles seem like 2."

*—Claire, age 42*
*Years running: 15*

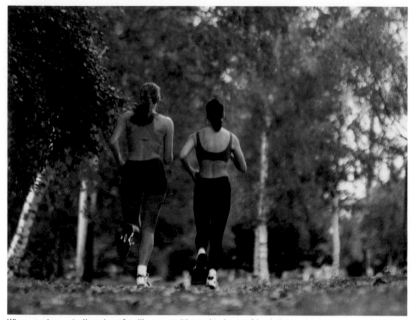

When running on trails or in unfamiliar areas, it's good to have a friend along.

a time when Paleolithic hunter-gatherers crossed great distances in groups. What worked for chasing down woolly mammoths works just fine when you're chasing fitness and endurance in today's sedentary society.

Some, if not most, group runs are organized by local running clubs, but some are pulled together by running shoe stores. In fact, chatting with the experienced staff at your local running shoe store is probably the most effective way of finding a group run.

Once you've found a group run, talk with or phone the run's organizer(s) about the composition of the group to get a sense of how you'll fit in. Group runs tend to center around a certain running pace, and if it's not yours, look elsewhere. The same goes for distance: If the group run is set for a distance farther than you've run in the past 2 weeks, keep looking, or simply put it off until you've reached that distance. Group runs should provide an opportunity to feel bolstered by others who enjoy running at your level; taking part in a run that leaves you way out front or lagging behind just won't reward you in any meaningful way. It makes sense to do your homework.

## JOIN A RUNNING CLUB

Of the two great elements about running clubs, one is obvious: You get a lot of running partners, and you're all in it together. The other benefit may surprise you: Many running clubs have coaches, and these individuals can have a profoundly beneficial impact on your performance.

Most running clubs offer one or more weekly runs, some with active coaching (meaning the coach runs with you) and some without (you all just show up at the appointed time and run together, without a coach). Some clubs center around a demographic group, such as women's clubs, or running clubs for seniors, whereas others are purely geographic in focus. If you live in a large city, you may be fortunate enough to have several from which to choose. If you find none, you can always start one yourself.

Running with a club gets you out exercising with others, and the social interaction is its own reward. You'll meet people with whom you share an obvious passion, and you'll likely create long lasting friendships. It's not all about the workout, either, since many clubs unwind after a run at local coffeehouses or pubs, or throw parties at other times for the pure fun of being together.

While you're imagining all the good times, let's return to the coach who's likely at the center of the club. In most, if not all cases, you'll get to know someone with years of running

## PAY YOUR DUES

Keep in mind that most clubs require members to pay modest annual dues, ranging anywhere from ten to thirty dollars. If you dislike the notion of paying dues, think of it this way. What you pay to join the running club will prevent you from buying the dozen pastries you might otherwise bring home from your local bakery on Saturday morning. When you consider what you might pay on a monthly basis for a gym membership (to say nothing of a personal trainer), a running club membership—with all the companionship, community, and running know-how you'll pick up from fellow members—is an absolute bargain.

at competitive levels. Depending on the size of the group, your opportunities for individual advice may be large or small, but you *will* learn a lot, both from the coach and your fellow club members. Join a running club and learn by osmosis—it can really happen.

## EXPLORE THE RUNNING WORLD ONLINE

The flip side of joining a local running club is connecting with a virtual network of runners at the click of a mouse. For starters, we suggest checking out the *Runner's World Forum* tab at *www.runnersworld.com*, then click on the "beginners" section. Cyber buddies abound, and you may very well hook up with some local runners that you found online. Want new options? Type "online running communities" or "online running forums" into your search engine and start exploring. Registering with a forum will give you rights to read other runners' posts, which can offer you a wealth of information. Read up, and if you feel like it, post your own questions, you're bound to get the answers you need. Forums are all the richer for the participation of many

people like yourself. You are bound to find plenty of personal advice. There are a lot of options on the Web, so you'll be spoiled for choice.

If you want a more personalized interaction, you can sign up with a virtual running coach. Open up your Internet browser, type "online running coaches" or simply "running coaches" into any search engine and check out the results. You'll have many options to peruse, from individual coaches to entire coaching organizations that offer services for runners, cyclists, and other athletes.

In many ways, virtual coaches offer more one-on-one attention than you'd get with the coach of your local club, with multiple phone conversations and e-mails a week. You'll get personalized weekly workouts and answers to all of your questions, and you'll get results: Most coaches say that their clients broaden the scope of their training, thanks to their coaches' expertise; this often leads to better running, both in and out of competition. All of these benefits do come with a cost, however, which varies with location and other factors.

# PART V:
# NEXT STEPS

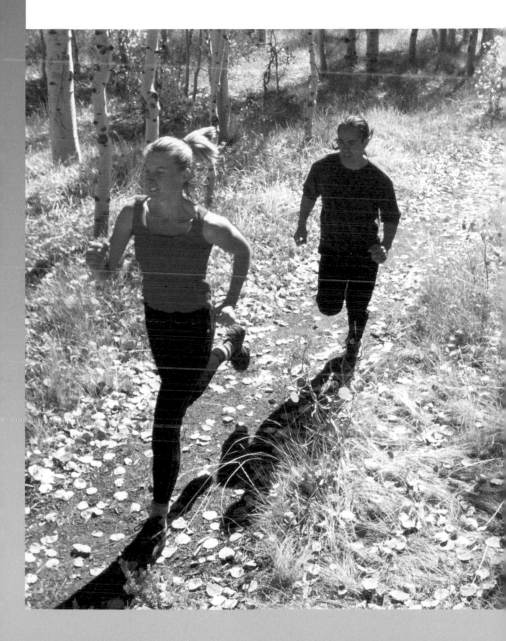

# Goals Will Get You There

Some people are natural goal-setters; if that describes you, you've already felt the power that striving for and achieving an ambition can create in your life. If you're not, don't worry. Despite the hundreds of goal-setting books out there, the practice is what you make it. The questions you ask yourself about running can clarify undeclared goals, or help you decide what's most important to you.

Take one of the simplest questions: Why are you running? How many of these answers are true for you? For weight loss; for stress reduction; for fitness and strength; to build endurance; to cross-train for another sport; for the community; for medical reasons; to fulfill a personal dream; for relaxation; for the competition; because someone said you could; because someone said you couldn't.

Were you surprised by your answers? You've completed the first step of identifying what's most important. On to the second step: Imagine yourself having achieved the goal, and work backwards to determine the steps you must take to accomplish that.

Set as many goals or as few as you like, but make sure they're yours. For example, don't get hung up on running because it's important to your significant other that you lose weight; include running in your life because losing weight, among other things, is important to you, and running will help you do it.

Thinking of your goals in terms of horizons for completion may help you to organize your efforts. You may wish to train for a 5-K race in a month, run a 7-minute mile in a year, and maintain the ability to run recreationally for the rest of your life. Once you have clarity as to the goal itself, how you'll achieve it, and its deadline, you need only concentrate on keeping yourself on the right track.

The final step in goal-setting is simple: Review your goals periodically to see what needs to

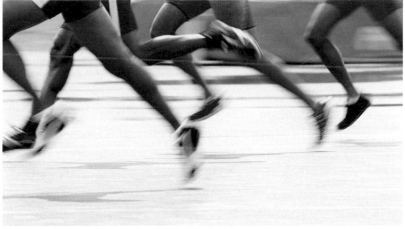

Having concrete goals will help you in your dash to the finish line.

change. Some objectives grow in importance over time, others diminish, and still others lose all importance in the face of new ones. Posing the important questions about running again and again will reconnect you with the motivation that got you started and keeps you going.

## KEEP A LOG

You've thought about your goals. You've imagined yourself achieving them. You've even started working out how to get there. The next step: Record it all in your training log.

If you've never kept a training log before, think of it as your running diary. It's for you alone to write or type in, scrutinize, and review as the pages fill up. What you include in your training log should allow you to record your runs, review your progress, and prepare for the future. That's past, present, and future—all in one place.

## RECORD THE PRESENT

The essential elements to include in your training log are: the date, time of day, and route of your run; how long you ran, the distance (if you know it), and your pace (again, if you know it); the type of workout you were engaged in (for instance, a weekly long run); how you felt about the run, and any other elements that seem important—"right knee hurts," for example. (For a sample entry, see the sidebar on page 81.)

At first, you may prefer to keep your log spare, getting to the heart of the matter without adding

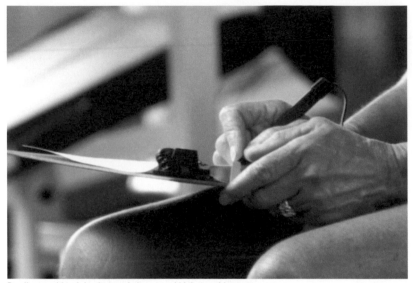

Reading an old training log can help you avoid injury and burnout.

a lot of fluff. Later, when you've built the habit of writing in your log, you may want to add information about the weather, how many miles you've put on your shoes, which shoes you wore, and (if you're a woman) where you are in your monthly cycle—as your log fills, this kind of information will help you see patterns in your running life. For instance, you may find that once the humidity creeps above 60 percent that your performance suffers.

Ideally, you will write in your log immediately after every run, when you'll remember all the details clearly. It's an excellent reward, and it also allows you closure on your workout.

## REVIEW THE PAST

Taking stock of your training on a weekly, monthly, and/or annual basis gives you a tremendous feeling of accomplishment—and vast amounts of valuable information. If you've been struggling with aches and pains, read through your log, keeping an eye out for patterns of overtraining and then think about changes you can make. Consider other important questions as well: Are you making progress, or are you stuck in a rut? How did you feel about your running? Are the mental images of your past runs motivating or do they leave you discouraged? Your answers to these questions can guide you toward your personal goals.

## >> A TRAINING LOG FOR EVERYONE

Training logs come in a variety of shapes, sizes and formats. Here's a list of easy-to-find options, from the fancy to the free:

- Program for your PDA that syncs up with a more complete application on your desktop.
- Off-the-shelf training log you can buy at the bookstore.
- Bound sketch book, with or without lines, available at bookstores and gift shops.

You're the boss, so buy or make the training log you want. Here's a sample entry to give you the hang of filling out your personal log.

| | |
|---|---|
| **Date:** April 3 | **Time:** 11:45 A.M. |
| **Route:** | Ocean trail |
| **Weather:** | Cool and breezy, about 50°F, low humidity |
| **Type of Run:** | Easy day |
| **Distance:** | 3 miles (1 mile timed, 2 miles @ 1 min. run/30 sec. walk), plus 10-min. warm-up and 5-min. cool-down. |
| **Comments:** | Felt great in the legs, but feet slapped the ground. Nailed the mile at 9:00 flat. No pain anywhere. |

## PLAN FOR THE FUTURE

If you're working through the 30/30 Plan or the 10-Week Run/Walk Plan, your workouts are pretty much figured out in advance. However, as you move beyond beginner status and into the realm of the intermediate runner, you'll need to start building your own weekly training plans that are commensurate with your goals. Whether in a graph, a computer spreadsheet, or simply as a handwritten list, sketch out what you're going to do during the week ahead. If you're feeling wiped out or unenthusiastic, build in more rest. Fatigue can mean that injuries are looming, so switch to easier workouts until your body has recovered. Be creative, use your judgment, and get feedback from more experienced runners as you need it.

# Start Cross-Training

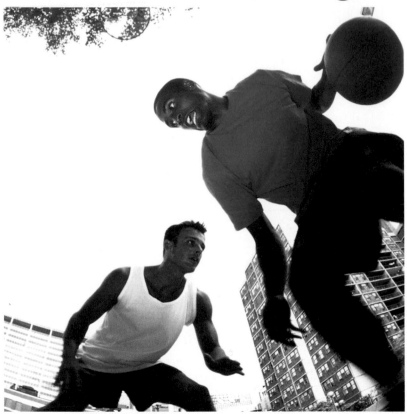

Working different muscles during different activities can prevent stress injuries.

**Cross-training is all about striking a balance. When you cross train, you balance the rigors of training in one sport with the rigors of another, or several. The result is that you, the athlete, are better prepared on a physical and mental level to excel.**

Running does a great job of working certain muscle groups including the hamstrings, your butt muscles (a.k.a. the glutes), and the calves, but leaves the quadriceps, the muscles on the front of your thighs, relatively undertaxed (and this is just one example). If you don't cross-train, this imbalance will make you more susceptible to injury over time, regardless of how conscientious you are about all the other aspects of training.

We've discussed the impact of running on joints, muscles, tendons, and ligaments, and the importance of getting your body used to this stress gradually. Ideally, you'll gravitate toward one or more cross-training sports that balance the benefits of running. Two of the best are cycling and swimming. Other options range from aerobics and hiking to martial arts to yoga.

## THE DOS AND DON'TS OF CROSS-TRAINING

There are right and wrong ways to incorporate cross-training into your life as a runner. Let's start with the right ways.

### DO:

**Cross train often** Train on your off days from running (though don't forgo a rest day to cross train), or after an easy run. However, be judicious about this second strategy; it's best employed when you have a strong fitness base.

**Work hard when you cross train** You're there to complement your running goals, so give it your all to get the best benefit.

**Cross train for 50 percent of your total workout time** As you begin your running career, take a look at the 30/30 and the 10-Week Run/Walk Plans and you'll see that walking accounts for at least half of the training time. After you grow stronger as a runner, you can replace more walking with cross-training.

### DON'T:

**Attempt to cross train in more than two sports** Don't overdo it, keep it simple and pick just one or two to focus on.

**Neglect proper form while cross-training** The time you invest in improving your swimming strokes, for example, will pay you back handsomely in enjoyment and improved performance.

**Let cross-training take over** The best way to excel at running is to do it, or put another way: No one ever became a champion runner by cycling all the time. Although it is important to cross-train, don't allow it to eclipse your focus on running.

Over the next several pages we present some basic training programs for two of the most popular cross-training sports for runners: swimming and cycling.

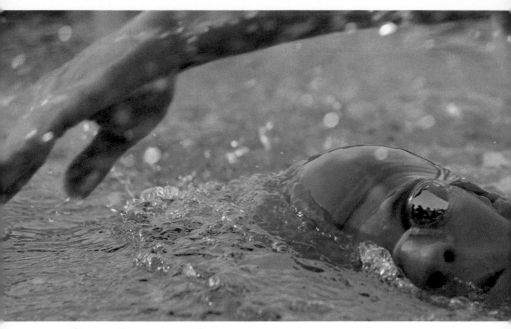

# Swimming

Swimming is a great cross-training sport for runners. Like running, swimming is a serious cardiovascular endeavor. Unlike running, swimming strengthens your shoulders, arms, core, and even your hips, while negating the effects of gravity and impact shock on your joints.

The combination of cool temperatures and water pressure helps relieve soreness by encouraging your muscles to eliminate waste products such as lactic acid. Swimming requires you to focus on proper form and promotes concentration and coordination—two skills that will serve you well as a runner.

Adapt this workout so that it best suits you: Remember, "hard" and "easy" are relative terms here. If you've been sedentary and are just starting out on your journey to fitness, it's better to take it slow. Rather than completing the entire workout, do as much as you are able to in 20 minutes. Another way to make the workout less strenuous—or for an assist if you're not the strongest swimmer—is to perform it using a kickboard.

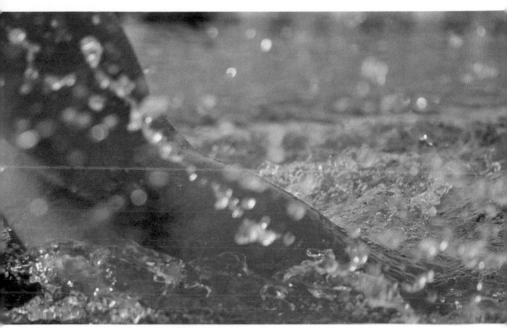
Swimming provides a low-impact total-body workout.

## LADDER WORKOUT

**Warm-up:** 250 yards at an easy pace
**Workout:**
- 25 yards easy, 25 yards hard, rest 20 seconds
- 25 yards easy, 50 yards hard, rest 20 seconds
- 50 yards easy, 75 yards hard, rest 20 seconds
- 75 yards easy, 50 yards hard, rest 20 seconds
- 25 yards easy, 25 yards hard, rest 20 seconds
- 25 yards easy

**Cool-down:** 100 yards at an easy pace
**Note:** Most pools in the U.S. are 25 yards long (22.9 m), whereas Olympic pools are 50 meters (54.7 yd) long; if an Olympic pool is your only option, swim widths.

# Cycling

If you're looking for a cross-training regimen that will improve your running, biking should be your choice. The motion of pedaling mimics the motion of running in such a way that it can improve your speed. In addition, cycling works the quadriceps, or quads, the large muscles on the front of the thigh—which running does little to strengthen.

Weak quads can cause or aggravate some common running injuries, including runner's knee and illiotibial band syndrome. Combine running with cycling, and the result is a balance in the strength of your leg muscles. Cycling works the legs, heart, and lungs without

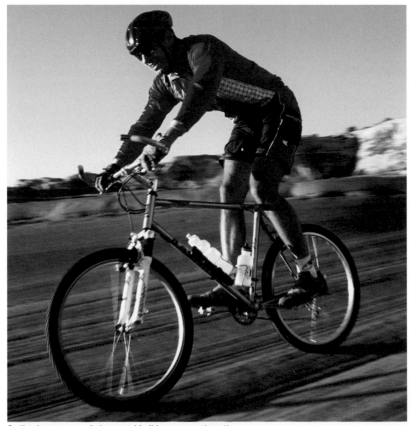

Cycling improves your balance and builds your core strength.

the joint impact of running, so it's well suited to runners who are recovering from certain types of injury. Cycling with a high spin cadence (pedaling at 80 to 90 revolutions per minute, also termed "spinning") will build the fast-twitch muscle fibers in your legs, which will allow you to stride faster while running.

## CYCLING WORKOUTS

There are a number of possible cycling workouts runners can do; here are just a few. No matter which you choose, make sure to take the time to pedal easily for 10 to 15 minutes to warm up.

**Workout one** Cycle for 30 minutes at a low gear on a flat course as a recovery workout on those days that you don't run. When you reach the point in your running career at which you're alternating hard and easy running days, you can just substitute this workout for an easy day. Just be careful not to overexert yourself as this would be counter productive.

**Workout two** Ride at a relaxed pace for between 1½ and 4 hours to build your endurance.

**Workout three** A 1-hour ride at a moderate effort will help an injured runner safely rebuild stamina and endurance.

Depending on your cross-training goals and your fitness level, you can choose to include additional elements. Keep in mind that these workouts are for intermediate to advanced runners, so don't feel pressured to rush into them.

**Hills** Hard climbs of 1½ to 3 minutes that force you to stand up out of the saddle will increase your stamina and push your muscles to the brink of fatigue, much like running sprints will.

**Hard/easy intervals** Hard cycling for 1 to 4 minutes followed by easy cycling for the same length of time will build speed and endurance. Repeat the cycle 1 to 3 times for a complete workout.

## I WISH I HAD KNOWN . . .

"It's important to build up your quadriceps muscles to protect your knees, especially before you try long runs or speed work."

—Marc, age 30
Years running: 10

# Stay Motivated

As a beginning runner, you may be grappling with a host of issues and that can present obstacles to maintaining a consistent training program. We discuss several of them here, suggest ways over, around, or through them, and better equip you to deal with them in the future.

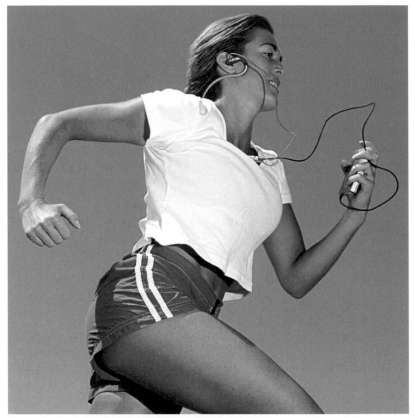

Everyone has tough days; the trick is to get through them.

**Too little time** A very common—and often illusory—roadblock. To find the time, use a calendar and book your running dates in advance. Penciling in an appointment to do your workout will motivate you to stick to it. You wouldn't cancel an important meeting or job interview, so don't back out of a run. Getting up 30 minutes earlier probably won't leave you exhausted, nor would running during your lunch break. You can even break up your runs into two parts—an A.M. and a P.M. portion. Running just a little is always better than not running at all.

**Feeling too full** If you consistently eat so much that you feel uncomfortably full, it's time to make a change. Eating small meals throughout the day is an effective way to avoid the bloated feelings that can be a de-motivating factor for any runner. Start a food diary to help you track how the "what" and "when" of your eating habits helps or hinders your running workouts.

**Too little sleep** Are your night-owlish habits wreaking havoc on your sleep cycle, leaving you too depleted to run? Give yourself some tough love and enforce a standard bedtime "window" every night. Maybe that means you turn off the lights each night between 9 and 10 P.M., or 10 and 11 P.M. Build in the flexibility you need so you won't rebel too strongly against a hard and fast number, but do inject a little discipline into your sleeping habits. Too little sleep can lead to burn out, loss of motivation, or injury. A warm glass of milk or reading something interesting—but not too exciting—before bed will also calm your jumpy mind and bring on those much needed *zzzs*.

## MUSIC WILL MOTIVATE YOU

We admit that running with headphones stirs debate among runners, many of whom believe that the music creates a distraction and makes a runner less attuned to their surroundings. But more runners than ever are listening to music on the go, thanks to lightweight and skip-proof MP3 players. Not only do runners say it clears the mind and psychs them up, but some scientific research suggests that listening to music during exercise actually stimulates certain areas of the frontal lobes, leading to post-workout improvements in cognitive function. If you do feel uneasy running outdoors with headphones, save them for the treadmill. You still have the mental boost you'll get after your run to look forward to.

**Too little energy** If you're coping poorly with periodic energy lows that threaten to derail your workout plans, eat a high-carbohydrate snack (a bagel or banana, for instance) an hour before your run to boost your blood sugar levels, and also within an hour afterwards (make sure this one has some protein as well). Caffeine may also help get you moving, but since it adds no real energy to your body, use it in moderation. If you're constantly feeling low, consult your physician or a sports nutritionist for tests that can help pinpoint what's ailing you.

**Bad weather** Rain, sleet, snow, hail, and the blazing heat of summer—they can really bring your motivation down. Protect yourself in advance with a trip to the sports clothing store, preferably one that specializes in running gear. If you shop in the off-season, you can stock up on appropriate gear at bargain prices. High-tech fabrics do a great job of protecting you from the elements.

**Too much running** Ahh, burnout. You recoil at the thought of even pulling on your socks. When enough is enough, you have several options, from saying no for a day or a week, to telling yourself that you're only going to do a fraction of your planned workout. Overtraining leads to injury, so heed the little voice in your head that's screaming at you to take it easy. You'll come back to running with renewed commitment. View your excuses as creative opportunities to problem-solve your situation, and you'll overcome them time after time.

## ENTER A RACE

After you've been running for a while, your beginner's enthusiasm will wane. Those first exultant weeks and months, during which your progress was exponential, will have passed, and you'll realize that for all the benefits of running, there is an investment required—no free lunch, in other words. Maybe you've even started to think of running as work—hard work. That's when you might want to consider entering a race.

Many runners enjoy their sport and never enter a race, and that's fine. However, we urge you to consider the idea. Racing provides runners with all sorts of benefits. It's often an opportunity for a new runner to discover what their actual pace is, since many races display measured mile markers along the course. Racing—especially in large events—allows

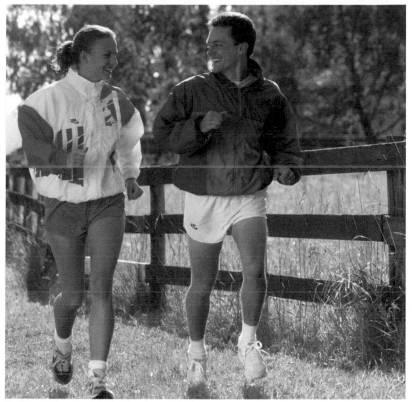

Finding a new route to run, or a running buddy, can often solve a case of low motivation.

beginners to run with other beginners and to discover that there will always be people out there who are faster, slower, taller, shorter, thinner, or heavier, but that they are all runners.

Here are some ways to dip your toes into the racing waters if you're still feeling a bit skittish about signing up.

**Join a fun run** Often these are family events for the benefit of a local institution like a library, church, or charitable cause. A fun run shares aspects of a race—it has a start and a finish—but the competitive aspects are downplayed in favor of a "hey, let's do this all together" spirit. Sign up and experience the community coming together, and run for the joy of it. Better yet, convince a training buddy to do it with you. Any anxiety you feel will dissipate with a friend at your side, and you may make new friends as well.

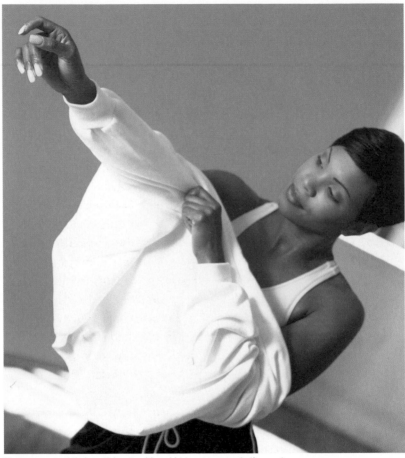

Most runs reward their participants with a shirt to commemorate the event.

**Sign up for a 5-K race** Once you've completed the 10-Week Run/Walk program, you're ready to start working toward your first race. The 5-K's low mileage (3.1 mi) makes it possible for novice runners to feel very confident of finishing, and usually draws large numbers of participants. Running in a bona fide race is fun, exciting, and awe-inspiring, and well worth your commitment. As with the fun run, consider doing the race with a training buddy.

**Go watch a race** We admit, there's no running involved, but rest assured that the experience of cheering on fellow runners will have a salutary effect on your own desire to get or remain involved with the sport and meet people who share your enthusiasm.

## TIPS FOR YOUR FIRST RACE

Go ahead and congratulate yourself for deciding to enter a race. Believe it or not, there are many runners whose anxiety about competition keeps them from ever doing what you've just done.

Preparing for your first race is all about ensuring that you enjoy yourself and want to sign up for another one afterwards. To that end, follow these simple tips:

**Check out the race site** If possible, visit the site and do a training run on the route a week or two beforehand, and get to know the course. Being comfortable with the route will calm some of your nervous energy.

**Eat familiar foods** The night before and the day of the race, stick to foods you know won't upset your stomach. This is not the time to branch out and try something that might not sit well with you during the race.

**Prepare well ahead** Get your race day gear—pre- and post-race snacks, drinks, and a change of clothes—ready the day before the race. You definitely don't want to be worried about this the morning of the race. It's also a good idea to pin your number on your shirt the night before the race.

However, if you don't pick up your number until the morning of the race, don't worry—safety pins will be provided and a volunteer will be glad to assist you in pinning on your racing bib.

**Hydrate** Sip water throughout the evening before and the morning of the race to ensure that you are well hydrated.

**Think positive thoughts** Professional athletes know the benefits of visualization. Imagine yourself the day of the race feeling confident, relaxed, and energetic.

**Sleep well** Try to get a good night's sleep before the race, but don't worry too much if nerves keep you awake—the sleep you get two nights before the race is even more important.

**Arrive early** Get to the race site early. Especially if it's a large event with lots of runners, you'll need time to go to the bathroom at least once, sign in and get your number (if you haven't already), check your bag (but not your valuables), find where you need to line up, and get in a good warm-up.

**Warm up** Keep your pre-race warm-up relaxed and easy: A mile of running (at the very most) or some walking, along with a few short striding lengths should warm your muscles sufficiently.

**Start slow—finish slow** During your first race, stay that way. Later, when you have more experience, you can increase your pace during the race. But for your first race, slow and steady is the key.

**Bring friends** Have family members and friends cheer you on at strategic points throughout the race. The boost you'll get from a supportive crowd is very real, so bring your own cheering squad.

**Know that it's okay to walk** Can't run the whole way? That's okay—especially during your first race, your goal should simply be to finish. If that means you need to take walk breaks, so be it; hold your head high as you cross the finish line.

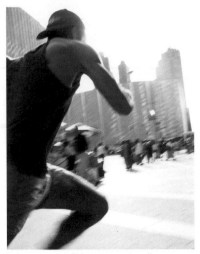

Being in a race will boost your adrenaline.

**Don't neglect your cool-down** The effort you've expended during a race makes cooling down more important than ever, so after you cross the finish line, keep it moving with a short walk.

## ›› NERVE TONIC

Butterflies in your stomach are completely normal, and deserve special attention. Since they're really just a reflection of your performance anxiety, try these strategies to quiet your nerves:

- Remind yourself that you're there to experience the race, and to enjoy yourself. Set aside your competitive ambitions for future races, focusing on finishing—not speed.
- Cultivate a feeling of connection with the other runners present. Regardless of individual goals, everyone is in it together, and the runners standing beside you feel, or have felt, the same emotions that you're feeling.
- Don't be afraid to talk to people. Telling stories and joking around with other runners will take your mind off yourself, and make you feel more relaxed and connected.